Wound Care

A Handbook for
Community Nurses

D1212345

Wound Care

A Handbook for Community Nurses

JOY RAINEY MSc, BSc, DPSN, RGN, DN
Tissue Viability Nurse, Wolverhampton Health Care

SERIES EDITOR
MARILYN EDWARDS, BSc(Hons), SRN, FETC
Specialist Practitioner, General Practice Nursing, Bilbrook Medical
Centre, Staffordshire

W
WHURR PUBLISHERS
LONDON AND PHILADELPHIA

© 2002 Whurr Publishers Ltd
First published 2002
by Whurr Publishers Ltd
19b Compton Terrace
London N1 2UN England and
325 Chestnut Street, Philadelphia PA 19106 USA

British Library Cataloguing in Publication Data

A catalogue record for this book
is available from the British Library.

ISBN 1 86156 289 6

Printed and bound in the UK by Athenaeum Press Ltd,
Gateshead, Tyne & Wear.

Contents

Series Preface

This series of handbooks has been devised to help community nurses answer commonly asked questions. Many of the questions are asked by patients, others by colleagues. The books have been written by specialists, and although they are not intended as full clinical texts, they are fully referenced from current evidence to validate the content. The purpose of each handbook is to provide 'facts at the fingertips', so that trawling through textbooks is not needed. This is achieved through the question and answer format, with cross-referencing between sections. Where further information may be required, the reader is referred to specific texts. Many patients want some control over their illnesses, and use the internet to access information. The useful address sections include website addresses to share with both patients and colleagues.

It is hoped that these handy reference books will answer most everyday questions. If there are areas which you feel have been neglected, please let us know for future editions.

Mandy Edwards

Preface

The day-to-day responsibility for wound management is usually undertaken by nurses. It includes assessing the wound, selecting an appropriate treatment and evaluating the patient's progress. To do this effectively the nurse needs to understand the healing process, recognise factors that may delay wound healing, understand how wound healing can be optimised, know how to recognise complications if they arise and know how to treat them. Only with a thorough understanding of these areas will it be possible to make a detailed assessment of the patient and the wound, and make a clinical decision on treatment that will be clinically effective.

Much of the success of wound care is built up from knowledge and experience, but inexperience of complications can leave the nurse unsure what to expect. This can be difficult to cope with, especially if the nurse works in an area where she has little peer support.

In recent years there have been numerous developments in wound management, and research has provided a better understanding of the healing process and how this can be optimised. Many new dressings have been developed and, although this should enhance wound management, the range available may make dressing selection a daunting task. Many factors affect dressing choice, including research articles, past experience, advice from colleagues and manufacturers' marketing strategies. The product chosen needs to be both efficacious and cost-effective.

This book is written for community nurses, including practice nurses who often work as the only nurse in a practice, which makes exchange of ideas and knowledge difficult. Some practice nurses see many wounds whereas others see wounds only rarely, so it is more difficult to build up a knowledge base on which to make clinical decisions. Nursing home nurses can also become isolated and may have difficulty getting release for study days.

The book aims to provide a picture of wound healing and related factors for both acute and chronic wounds that may be encountered in a community practice situation. An overview of the function of the skin and phases of wound healing is given before looking at the relationship between wound healing and the patient's health and lifestyle. Wound assessment is an essential component for wound management. This is discussed in detail in Chapter 2. There are many dressing types available to community nurses, and Chapter 5 guides the reader through the uses of commonly used products.

The question and answer format includes many of the questions frequently asked by nurses. Case studies are also used to give examples of both good and bad practice.

Finally, I would like to express my sincere gratitude to Sarah Freeman, BA(Hons), Clinical Governance Coordinator, Wolverhampton Primary Care Groups, for her contribution of Chapter 12.

Joy Rainey
September 2001

CHAPTER 1

Wound healing

This chapter is a basic examination of the functions of the skin, how wounds can be categorised, the stages and mechanisms of wound healing, and how a moist environment enhances wound healing. To understand these processes in greater depth, it would be necessary to consult a detailed anatomy and physiology text.

Q1.1   What functions does the skin have?

The skin is the largest organ of the body. It covers approximately 2 m² and weighs around 3 kg. The skin has many functions, which include the following:

- Maintenance of body temperature
- Protection from bacteria, dehydration, ultraviolet radiation and physical abrasion
- Presence of nerve endings that warn of unpleasant stimuli such as pain and extreme heat
- Helping the body gain vitamin D from sunlight.

Q1.2   What problems occur when the skin is broken?

Once the skin is broken the protective functions of the skin are lost. The greater the skin loss the more serious these problems will be.

Bacteria and other micro-organisms can gain entry into deeper tissues and cause infection (see Q10.1 and Q10.2). Fluid is lost from the body and if the area of skin lost is large enough (as in a major burn) this can be life threatening.

Q1.3   How is the skin made up?

The skin is made up from two layers: the outer epidermis and the dermis. The dermis contains hair follicles, sebaceous glands and sweat glands. Beneath the dermis is subcutaneous fatty tissue containing nerves, blood vessels and lymphatics (Figure 1.1).

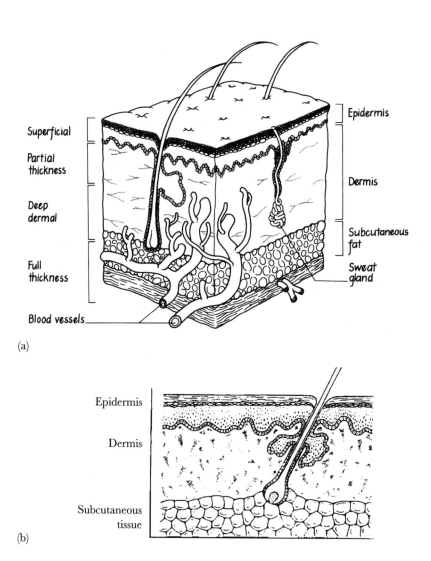

Figure 1.1 The skin.

Q1.4   Can I tell by looking at a wound what layers are damaged?

Superficial wounds damage only the epidermis (Figure 1.2). If the dermis is intact, normal skin markings will be present. Partial-thickness wounds damage the dermis and will look pale pink (Figure 1.3). Full-thickness wounds reach the subcutaneous fatty tissue or go deeper to muscle and bone (Figure 1.4). These wounds may reveal islands of yellow fat and may expose muscle, tendon or bone.

Q1.5   What is the definition of a wound?

A wound is an abnormal break in the skin, as the result of cell death or damage.

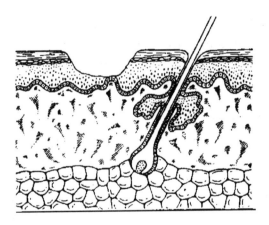

Figure 1.2 A superficial wound.

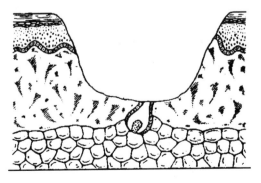

Figure 1.3 A partial-thickness wound.

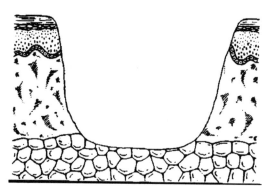

Figure 1.4 A full-thickness wound.

Q1.6   How are wounds described or categorised?

Wounds are often put into different categories or classifications. This enables professionals to share information and experiences knowing that they are talking about similar wounds. Wounds can be classified in several ways but each wound is unique and deserves individual care.

Primary or secondary intention

A common way of classifying wounds is by differentiating between those that heal by primary or secondary intention (see Q1.7).

Those healing by primary intention are those with skin edges that have been brought together, usually by sutures, clips, adhesive strips or surgical adhesive. These may be traumatic lacerations or surgical wounds.

Secondary intention describes wound healing when the skin edges are not brought together, and have to heal by contracting and filling up with granulation tissue. These wounds include leg ulcers, pressure damage, and lacerations with substantial tissue loss or dirty surgical or traumatic injuries, which may become infected if the skin edges are opposed and secured.

Types of tissue

Wounds can also be categorised by the type of tissue within the wound:

- The wound contains black necrotic tissue (see Q2.10)
- The wound is yellow and sloughy (see Q2.11)

- The wound is red and granulating (see Q2.12)
- The wound is starting to display signs of the formation of new pink epithelial tissue (see Q2.13)
- The wound is green and infected (see Q2.14).

Depth of wound

Wounds can also be classified by depth. This is a common way of describing pressure sores and several scales exist. An example of this is the UK consensus classification of pressure sore severity (Stirling scale; Reid and Morison 1994) (Table 1.1).

Although it is not usual to see pressure sores in the general practitioner's surgery, this type of classification can be used or adapted to describe other wounds. Also, although these are the most common ways of categorising wounds, other methods can be used, such as by the cause or by the stage of the healing process that the wound has reached.

Table 1.1 The UK consensus classification of pressure sores

Stage 1	Discoloration of intact skin (light finger pressure applied to the intact skin does not alter the discoloration)
Stage 2	Partial-thickness skin loss or damage involving epidermis and/or dermis
Stage 3	Full-thickness skin loss involving damage or necrosis of subcutaneous tissue but not extending to underlying bone, tendon or joint capsule
Stage 4	Full-thickness skin loss with extensive destruction and tissue necrosis extending to underlying bone, tendon or joint capsules

Q1.7   What do the terms 'primary' and 'secondary intention' mean?

As previously mentioned, wounds can be described as healing by primary or secondary intention (see Q1.6). Healing by primary intention should be achieved for all incised surgical wounds and primary closed lacerations. Wound healing should be rapid because there is no tissue loss and the skin edges are held together (see Q1.6).

In wounds healing by secondary intention, the wound edges are apart and the defect will need to fill with granulation tissue before new epidermis can cover the wound. These include leg ulcers, open incisions (e.g. after draining abscesses when closure may encourage infection) and full-thickness burns.

Occasionally, wounds may be described as healing by tertiary intention. This is desirable if the wound, such as a laceration, has been contaminated, e.g. dirt following an accident. The wound is initially cleaned and left open. If there appears to be little risk of infection it is then closed in the normal way (Dealey 1994).

 Q1.8 What are the phases of wound healing?

Wound healing is usually described in four physiological phases: the inflammatory, destructive, proliferative and maturation stages (Professional Development 1994). In reality it is a continuous process with the stages merging and overlapping.

The inflammatory stage: 0–3 days (Figure 1.5)

When tissue is injured or disrupted the body's immediate response is to re-establish haemostasis. Damaged cells and blood vessels release histamine, causing vasodilatation of the surrounding capillaries, taking serous exudate and white cells to the area of damage.

 It is this increased blood flow and serous exudate that cause local oedema, redness and heat, giving rise to an inflamed appearance.

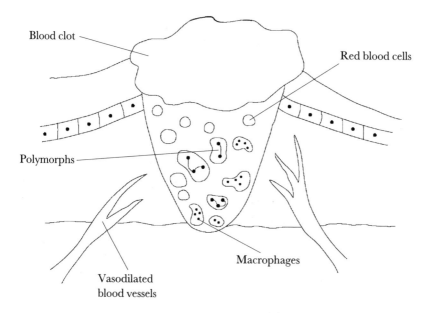

Figure 1.5 The inflammatory stage: 0–3 days.

The coagulation system and platelets cause the blood to clot, which prevents further bleeding or loss of body fluids. Injured vessels thrombose and red cells become entangled in a fibrin mesh, which begins to dry and becomes a scab. The scab is the body's natural defence to keep out micro-organisms. Phagocytic white cells (polymorphs and macrophages) are attracted to the area to defend against bacteria, ingest debris and begin the process of repair. In a clean acute wound this stage lasts up to 3 days. If the wound is infected or necrotic tissue is present this stage is prolonged.

Destructive phase: 1–6 days (Figure 1.6)

White cells line the walls of blood vessels and migrate through the walls, which become more porous, into surrounding tissue. Here phagocytic cells break down devitalised necrotic tissue, and the macrophages engulf and ingest bacteria and dead tissue. In addition, the macrophages stimulate the development of new blood vessels and the formation and multiplication of fibroblasts, which in turn are responsible for the synthesis of collagen and other connective tissues. This stage normally lasts from 1 to 6 days, but white cell activity can be compromised in dry exposed wounds (Morison 1991).

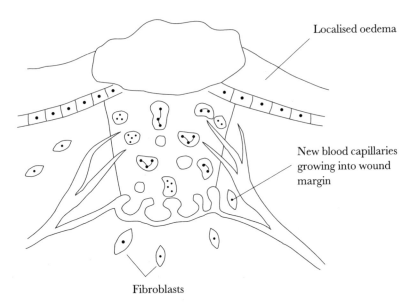

Localised oedema

New blood capillaries growing into wound margin

Fibroblasts

Figure 1.6 The destructive stage: 1–6 days.

Proliferative phase: 3–24 days (Figure 1.7)

The fibroblasts continue to multiply, forming collagen fibrils, which make a fibrous network. This traps red blood cells, which go on to become new capillary loops. At this stage the tissue is very delicate, having none of the organisation of normal tissue. This granulation tissue is so called because of its red granular appearance. As the collagen matures, there is a rapid increase in the tensile strength. Signs of inflammation subside and the process of contraction begins. In an open wound, this stage may be prolonged because more collagen is needed to repair the tissue defect.

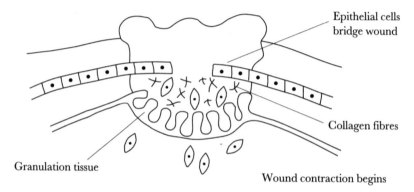

Figure 1.7 The proliferative stage: 3–24 days.

Maturation phase: 24 days to 1 year (Figure 1.8)

When the wound has filled with granulation tissue, collagen fibres pull in the wound, causing it to contract and become smaller. This speeds up the healing process as less collagen will be necessary to repair the defect. As the wound space decreases, vascularity also decreases, fibroblasts shrink and the collagen fibres change the red granulation tissue to white avascular tissue as epithelium migrates inwards. Epithelial cells will migrate from the wound edge, sweat glands and the remnants of hair follicles. They migrate over the granulation tissue until they meet with like cells from another area of the wound, sometimes forming islands in the wound centre. This process is slowed down if the wound is dry and has a scab or eschar over it (see Q2.10). In this case they have to burrow under the dry scab (see Q1.9). Migrating cells lose their ability to divide and so

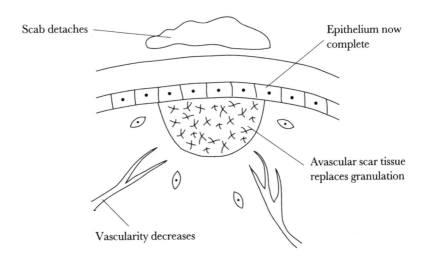

Scab detaches

Epithelium now
complete

Avascular scar tissue
replaces granulation

Vascularity decreases

Figure 1.8 The maturation stage: 24 days to 1 year.

epithelialisation depends on the ability of like cells to keep meeting. When the surface of the wound is covered with epithelial cells, the epithelium thins. Hair follicles are not replaced. Wound maturation usually takes between 24 days and 1 year.

Q1.9   What is meant by moist wound healing?

Traditionally, wound care encouraged nurses to allow wounds to dry out and form a scab. This was thought to provide a mechanical barrier to infection and be the most appropriate treatment. Extensive research has shown that this is not the case (although some clinicians and many patients still cling to traditional methods).

Work on moist wound healing started in the early 1960s. The most quoted research in relation to this is Winter (1962) who conducted a clinical trial using superficial wounds on pigs. Half of these wounds were allowed to dry out and form scabs, whereas the other half were covered with polythene, thus creating a moist environment. The results showed that those covered with polythene epithelialised nearly twice as fast as those wounds allowed to dry out. After examining the histology, Winter concluded that, in the dry wounds, epithelial cells were handicapped when migrating across the wound surface by the collagen fibres joining the scab to the surface of the wound. Epithelial cells in the moist wounds could migrate more quickly through the wound exudate and did not need to traverse a scabbed area (see Q2.13).

Dyson et al. (1988) have shown that a moist wound moves through the inflammatory stage of healing faster than a dry wound and produces greater capillary growth.

Initially it was thought that the moist environment may encourage greater bacterial growth and lead to a higher number of wound infections. This view has been disproved. Studies by Hutchinson and Lawrence (1991) showed that the reverse was true and occluded wounds showed a lower rate of infection.

Since the late 1970s, manufacturing companies have been creating dressings that give a moist environment to speed wound healing. Some clinicians who cling to traditional products, such as gauze, use the higher cost of modern products to support their choice. However, modern products encourage wounds to heal faster and get infected less often. The unit cost becomes less relevant when viewed in relation to patient discomfort (see Q2.7), nursing time and greater use of other materials, such as sterile gloves, aprons, dressing packs and antibiotics.

Summary

The skin is a large organ with many functions. Wounds can be categorised in several ways, which enables standardisation of classification throughout the nursing profession.

Wounds can heal by primary, secondary or tertiary intention, with wound healing occurring in several phases. In reality this is a continuous process with stages overlapping. It has been well established that wounds granulate better when kept moist.

CHAPTER 2
Wound assessment

Wound assessment is a vital part of wound care if the healing process is to be optimised. This chapter discusses the information that needs to be sought and documented to complete a wound assessment, and explains why documentation is important both for reasons of practical/clinical effectiveness and as a legal and professional requirement.

Q2.1 Why is it important to assess a wound thoroughly?

Wound assessment is commonly a responsibility left to the nurse. For the care given to be appropriate, it is important that this is done thoroughly to identify a goal of treatment; for example this may be to deslough, to protect and keep moist, to choose the most appropriate treatment, and to evaluate treatment to check for progress or deterioration. It is also important that this assessment and subsequent evaluations are clearly documented, for several reasons. First, it allows evaluation to take place. If good records are not kept, the evaluation is likely to be vague and subjective with reliance on comments such as 'looking better' or 'healing well', which say nothing about the state of the wound. This is perhaps even more important if more than one person is responsible for the patient's care. Second, records are of extreme importance in case of complaint or litigation. In legal terms, if it is not recorded, the care did not happen, so records must be timely, accurate and clear (see Q2.2).

Although assessment may seem a lengthy process, the time spent assessing a wound should lead to the selection of appropriate treatment. This should optimise wound healing and lead to swifter resolution of care.

Thorough assessment of the wound will take time, but if it leads to the correct treatment being chosen and wound healing optimised it is time well spent. In the longer term, the patient requires fewer episodes of care. Assessment details can be written in the patient notes or on a purpose-made chart. An example is shown in Figure 2.1.

Patient name: Ann Jones Type of wound: Laceration	Position of wound: Left shin Duration of wound: 2 weeks			
Date	1/6/00			
Size of wound:				
Maximum width	3 cm			
Maximum length	1 cm			
Type of tissue within wound:				
e.g. slough, necrosis, granulation	Granulation			
Exudate:				
Amount, colour	Minimal			
Odour:				
None, some, offensive	None			
Pain				
Where, when, severity	Occasionally if touched			
Surrounding skin:				
Erythema, wet/dry, eczema	Healthy			
Infection:				
Suspected, swab taken, result	Not clinically indicated			
Treatment summary:				
Cleansing lotion, if used	None			
Topical treatment to wound and surrounding skin	None			
Primary dressing	Duoderm			
Secondary dressing	None			
Fixed by	N/A			
Assessed by	ME			

Figure 2.1 An example of a wound assessment chart.

Q2.2   The nurse only has about 10 minutes to see each patient. Wouldn't a brief note be sufficient?

Records must be kept in order to aid clinical decision-making (Williams 1997) (see Q2.1). The UKCC Professional Code of

Conduct (UKCC 1992) states that one of the purposes of records maintained by the registered nurse is to 'provide a base line record against which improvement or deterioration can be judged'. The importance of clear concise records and the failure to maintain them can be seen as a negligent act and a breach of a nurse's duty to care (Moody 1993).

To illustrate this point consider the following scenario.

Scenario for case study 1

Nurse S had seen Fred on his first visit to the surgery with a leg ulcer. She performed a full assessment, including Doppler recordings, and diagnosed the ulcer to be the result of arterial insufficiency. Fred drank about four times the recommended alcohol limit each week and admitted to smoking about 40 cigarettes a day. He also had poorly controlled type 1 diabetes and a history of heart problems.

Nurse S clearly remembered her discussion with Fred and strongly suggested that he reduce his alcohol and cigarette consumption and modify his diet. She also verbally recommended to the GP that a vascular opinion was required. However, after performing the assessment, she was running late and the entry in her records reported 'Doppler shows arterial, advice given'.

Over the next few weeks, the ulcer continued to deteriorate and Fred's approach to life remained the same. Nurse S remembered talking to Fred repeatedly about his lifestyle and diabetes. Her records stated 'Looks larger', 'Redressed', 'Larger, advice given'.

Fred received his appointment for a vascular assessment but 4 weeks before this he developed a severe infection in his leg. This required immediate admission and resulted in below-knee amputation.

His family complained to the health authority about Fred's care and said the amputation was the result of the care he received by the practice nurse. They stated that Fred was unaware that his alcohol consumption, smoking and diabetes could result in amputation.

From her records could you defend her practice?

Q2.3   What should be included in a wound assessment?

It is important that the cause of the wound is identified and recorded. Personal observation suggests that acute wounds such as lacerations, bites and postoperative wounds are usually clearly identified, but chronic wounds such as leg ulcers are generalised. It is important that the exact underlying cause is identified. Is it a venous ulcer (see Q8.5 and Q8.6)? Is it an arterial ulcer (see Q8.7–Q8.9)? Did the wound start from trauma or a bite? In this case there may be no underlying disease.

The treatment for each wound type is different and, in the case of venous and arterial ulcers the opposite, so without identification the chosen treatment may be incorrect. Leg ulcers are discussed in more detail in Chapter 8.

Position

The position of the wound should be clearly documented and may be aided by the use of diagrams.

Size

The size of the wound should be recorded (see Q2.4).

History

The history of the wound should be taken. Ask the patient how long it has been present, who, up until now, has been dressing it and what treatments have been used. This will give some indication of any allergies or treatments that have previously failed. The wound may be a recurrence of a leg ulcer (particularly venous) and treatment of previous episodes of ulceration may be relevant (see Q8.32).

Skin condition

It is important to assess the surrounding skin. Any redness or erythema may indicate infection. If the patient has fragile skin, perhaps caused by medication such as long-term steroid use, it may be inappropriate to apply an adhesive dressing.

Leg ulcers may be surrounded by varicose eczema, which may require an emollient, or by contact dermatitis from previous treatments, which may require a short course of a topical steroid cream (see Q5.20, Q8.14 and Q8.26).

Tissue

The state of the tissue within the wound should be recorded. This will help to identify the goal of treatment and in many ways identify an appropriate treatment. There may be more than one type of tissue within the wound in which case an estimate of the percentage of each type should be made, e.g. 30% slough, 70% granulation (see Q2.11 and Q2.12).

Pain

The patient's level of pain should be assessed and treated with appropriate analgesia. Other factors to consider are:

- Is the pain ischaemic? (see Q8.8 and Q8.9)
- Is the wound infected? (see Q10.1)
- Is the dressing causing pain either by drying out and adhering to the wound surface, or by causing an allergic reaction? (see Q8.26 and Q8.27)
- Is the wound painful at dressing change because the dressing has dried out or is being removed inappropriately? (see Q2.7)

Any wound odour should also be recorded. This may be a sign of infection, or may be anaerobes in necrotic tissue (see Q2.6).

Q2.4 How should wounds be measured?

It is important to record wound size so that healing progress or deterioration can be observed. Both the nurse and patient can be motivated if healing can be observed. This also encourages the patient's compliance with continuing a treatment about which they are not enthusiastic, such as compression therapy (see Q8.29).

The simplest way to record wound size is to take the maximum dimensions with a ruler (Figure 2.2). A more accurate way is to trace the wound, using a purpose-made chart (available from several companies that manufacture dressings), acetate sheets or the clear packaging in which many dressings come. The tracing can be either stored in the patient's notes or used as a template to draw around and add to notes. Consider whether or not the plastic is sterile. It is advisable to hold non-sterile materials slightly above the wound surface or to cleanse the surface touching the wound both before and afterwards with an Alcowipe.

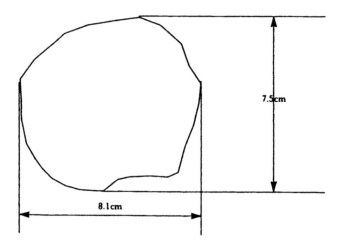

Figure 2.2 Measuring a wound.

Photographs are the most accurate way to record size and appearance of large wounds (see Q2.5). Wound depth can be more difficult to measure, but use of a sterile probe is probably the most accurate method. These are sometimes available from pharmaceutical companies.

Q2.5   What sort of issues must be considered when purchasing a camera?

Perhaps the most important issue is informed patient consent. If the materials are to be used for teaching or publication this consent should be written. There are several other issues to consider before embarking on wound photography. Bellamy (1995) suggests the following:

* Choice of equipment
* Choice of materials
* Choice of processing
* Control of subject
* Control of lighting
* Control of background.

Equipment in the main may be what is affordable. Many people choose a Polaroid-type camera because they get instant results and they do not have to worry about where to get material processed or finishing a whole film. Results, however, may not be as good as with a 35-mm single-lens reflex camera.

With the choice of materials, because the colour of a wound is an important indicator of condition, only colour film should be used (Bellamy 1995). If the pictures are to be stored in patients' notes, prints are adequate, but if photographs are to be used for publication or teaching purposes, slides may be more practical.

Thought should be given to processing. High-street 'quick process' shops may have photographs rotating behind the counter. Local labs may even have someone working there who recognises the patient. The use of a geographically distant professional laboratory that can provide confirmation of confidentiality is recommended (Bellamy 1995.) Films should be hand transferred (e.g. by courier) or if necessary sent by registered post, but not by regular mail. Put a ruler close to the wound so that the size can be roughly ascertained. This will aid reassessment and show progress. It is also useful to write the date and the patient's initials on a piece of adhesive tape and stick this close to the wound; this helps to identify the patient and also to place photographs in chronological order.

Lighting may be difficult to control in a surgery or within the patient's home and most nurses are not expert photographers. A flash or a camera with an automatic flash will be necessary in most cases. The background to any clinical photograph should be plain and unobtrusive rather than the clutter of a dressing trolley, treatment room, kitchen or front room.

Once taken and developed, photographs form part of a patient's clinical records and should be stored with the same care.

Q2.6   What can be done about wound odour?

Odour can be very distressing for the patient and often occurs in heavily infected or fungating wounds (see Q11.1). Personal experience shows that this may be the only reason a patient has sought treatment. Some dressings such as hydrocolloids may cause odour when they interact with wound exudate (see Q5.16). If this is expected to happen, either at dressing change or if the dressing leaks, it is worth reassuring the patient that the wound has not become infected.

Charcoal dressings may be used to absorb odour (see Q5.23). Oral or topical metronidazole may reduce wound odour (Ashford et al. 1984; Newman et al. 1989), or an aromatherapy oil of the patient's choosing may be applied to the outer dressing.

Q2.7   What points should be considered in regard to pain?

Pain is a subjective experience arising within the brain in response to damage to body tissues (Bond 1984). It is an issue that is often overlooked in wound care. Pain perception is unique to each individual and subjective (McCaffery 1983). Pain is what the patient says it is. Nurses' interpretation of a patient's pain will affect the care that is given (Hoskins and Welchew 1985).

Differing wounds will result in different types of pain. Skin damage results in pain that is often described as 'cutting' or 'burning'. This usually responds well to non-steroidal anti-inflammatory drugs (Emflorgo 1999). If blood vessels are injured, pain may be described as 'throbbing' in nature. If long-term ischaemia is a likely outcome, opiate analgesia may be required; if this is unlikely it may be required initially and then reduced (Emflorgo 1999). Damage to nerves results in itching, tingling, smarting or stinging. This may respond to anti-epileptic drugs (Bond 1984; Warfield 1997). Studies also show that a moist wound healing environment, which bathes nerve endings in fluid, prevents their stimulation and thus reduces discomfort (Thomas 1990) (see Q1.9). Occlusive dressings that produce an anaerobic environment also reduce wound pain (Johnson 1988). If a wound dries out or the dressing causes drying at the surface, localised pain results. This can happen if polysaccharide bead dressings or alginate dressings are applied to lightly exuding wounds (Thomas 1990) (see Q5.9–Q5.10).

Pain on dressing removal can occur if the dressing becomes incorporated into the wound. Newly formed capillaries may grow into dressings with mesh surfaces (Dealey 1994), or if the dressing becomes saturated with exudate and then dries and adheres to the wound surface (Value for Money Unit 1997) (see Q5.5). In these situations wound pain occurs and damage occurs to tissue at each dressing change. Soaking the dressing off is time-consuming and does not always result in pain-free removal (Thomas 1990).

Infection is associated with pain, so check the wound for the signs of infection (Cutting and Harding 1994) (see Q10.1) and treat with systemic antibiotics if infection is present. Pain also occurs as a result of poor bandage technique, which causes bandage slippage, or has insufficient padding or incorrect application (see Q8.29).

Venous leg ulcers are often said to be not painful unless accompanied by oedema or infection; however, Hofman et al. (1997) reported that 64% of patients experienced pain. Arterial leg ulcers often cause severe and persistent pain, which may require treatment with opiates (see Q8.9).

Pain from pressure ulcers depends on the depth of the wound. Deep ulcers often result in less severe pain than shallow ones because the nerve endings in the skin have been destroyed (Emflorgo 1999). However, if the area is swollen or infected, pain is likely. As with pressure ulcers, small deep burns often result in a lower level of pain than more superficial ones, but the site of the burn is significant. Those to the hands, face or genitalia are more painful.

Q2.8   How should pain be assessed?

Accurate pain assessment is the key to pain relief. Nurses often fail to use even a simple assessment tool. A visual analogue scale is a practical tool for assessing a patient's pain at dressing changes (Choiniere et al. 1990). Type and amount of pain vary between individuals; studies have shown that nurses often fail to believe patients' reports of pain (Saxey 1986; Seers 1987). An example of a pain assessment scale is shown in Figure 2.3.

Q2.9   How should pain be managed?

Appropriate analgesia should be offered following liaison with the GP, but other measures should also be taken.

A dressing should be chosen that will not stick to the wound and cause trauma, and that is right for the exudate level, keeps the wound moist and allows pain-free removal.

Cleansing should be by gentle irrigation with warm physiological saline (see Q4.2–Q4.4) if it is necessary to remove debris.

Wounds should not be rubbed or scrubbed; this will not only cause unnecessary pain but will also damage the wound bed.

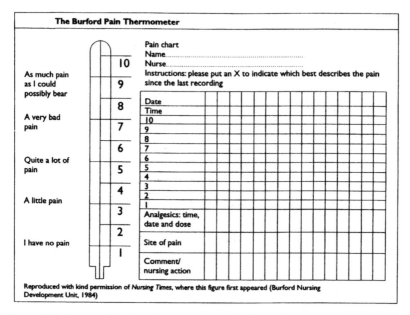

The Burford Pain Thermometer

As much pain as I could possibly bear	10
	9
A very bad pain	8
	7
	6
Quite a lot of pain	5
	4
A little pain	3
	2
I have no pain	1

Pain chart
Name...
Nurse...
Instructions: please put an X to indicate which best describes the pain since the last recording

Date																					
Time																					
10																					
9																					
8																					
7																					
6																					
5																					
4																					
3																					
2																					
1																					
Analgesics: time, date and dose																					
Site of pain																					
Comment/ nursing action																					

Reproduced with kind permission of *Nursing Times*, where this figure first appeared (Burford Nursing Development Unit, 1984)

Figure 2.3 An example of a pain assessment scale. Reproduced by kind permission of Nursing Times where this first appeared, 9 May 1984, Vol 80, No 19, p. 58.

Other therapies such as relaxation techniques, heat and cold therapies, and diversion therapy can all help reduce perceived pain (Emflorgo 1999).

Q2.10 What is necrotic tissue and how should it be treated?

A wound may contain necrotic tissue, which may be soft, spongy and black/grey, or form a hard black eschar over the wound surface. It is the result of tissue death secondary to ischaemia. This will always delay healing and increases the chance of wound infection. The treatment aim will be débridement by use of an appropriate dressing (see Q5.11 and Q5.15), or if necessary seeking a surgical opinion on sharp débridement when tissue is surgically removed.

Q2.11 What is slough and how should it be treated?

Yellow or sloughy tissue is formed in many chronic wounds. It is not dead tissue but a mixture of dead cells and serous exudate. It needs to be removed to optimise healing and is a similar process to débridement (see Q5.15 and Q5.16). It is important not to mistake exposed tendons or epithelial islands for slough because they can have a similar appearance.

Q2.12 What is granulation tissue and how should it be treated?

Red or granulating wounds have fragile new tissue forming, which is easily damaged. The aim of treatment will be to protect the tissue and provide a moist environment to optimise healing (see Q1.9). Particular care should be taken during wound cleansing (see Q4.1–Q4.4) and a dressing should be selected that will not adhere to the surface of the wound and cause trauma during dressing changes.

Q2.13 What is epithelial tissue and how should it be treated?

Pink or epithelial tissue is the new layer of epidermis, which will cover the wound when it has filled up with granulation tissue. The epithelial cells migrate from the wound margins. They sometimes meet to form clusters or islands on the wound surface. A moist environment aids movement of these cells, so the chosen dressing should again provide this environment and protect the wound surface (see Q1.9).

Q2.14 How do I recognise an infected wound?

The classic symptoms of wound infection include the following:

- Erythema
- Oedema
- Increased exudate
- Offensive odour
- Pain
- Pyrexia.

See Q10.1–Q10.4, Q10.7 and Q10.13 for more details on recognising and treating wound infection.

Summary

Thorough assessment of all wounds is a prerequisite for good care. Allowing the patient to see progress improves motivation and compliance; wound measurement is simple and does not require special skills. The wound should be treated in relation to the tissue state within the wound. This will change over time and regular reassessment is needed. Assessment and treatment of pain are important parts of wound care. Record keeping is a legal and professional requirement and accurate documentation is essential.

CHAPTER 3

Factors affecting wound healing

It is not only the dressing that is chosen which affects the way wounds heal. This chapter examines other issues that may impact on wound healing, and explains why it is important to look at the patient's lifestyle and health status when assessing the patient and planning his or her wound management.

Q3.1   What should be included in a general assessment of the patient?

As well as assessing the wound itself, it is important to look at the patient holistically. Many factors influence wound healing. If these are not addressed, healing will be delayed or may even fail to take place. Some of the factors affecting healing are listed in Table 3.1. Not all can be treated but, if highlighted, at least an understanding of why healing is slow can be reached.

Table 3.1 Factors affecting wound healing

Age	See Q3.2, Q9.4
Concurrent disease	See Q3.3, Q9.4
Nutritional status	See Q3.4–Q3.7, Q9.4
Drugs	See Q3.8, Q9.4
Smoking	See Q3.9
Excessive alcohol consumption	See Q3.10
Mobility	See Q9.4, Q8.14

Q3.2   What effect does age have on wound healing?

As people age the metabolic processes slow down, which prolongs tissue repair. Wound infection may also be more common as immune competence becomes less specific and inflammation less effective (David 1986) (see Q10.2). Elderly people are more likely to have chronic concurrent illness, which may delay healing and require drug therapy.

Q3.3   Which concurrent diseases particularly interfere with wound healing?

- Diabetes has long been associated with poor wound healing. It is important to control diabetes if wound healing is to be achieved. People with diabetes are also more susceptible to wound infection (see Q8.18).
- Cardiovascular and pulmonary disease may delay wound healing because the transport of oxygen to the wound site may be inadequate, and oxygen is essential for wound healing (see Q3.9).
- Uraemia increases the risk of wound dehiscence as a result of a reduction in collagen deposition. Granulation may also be delayed (see Q1.8).
- Thyroid or pituitary deficiency may delay healing as a result of slowed metabolic rates.
- Cushing's syndrome treated with steroids will delay healing (see Q3.8).
- Rheumatoid arthritis often necessitates high doses of corticosteroids (see Q8.16).

Q3.4   How does diet affect wound healing?

Both obesity and malnourishment inhibit wound healing. Advice from a community dietitian may be needed in some cases.

Poor nutrition and malnourishment adversely affect wound healing in many ways. The links between nutrients and healing are shown in Table 3.2. It should be remembered that injury may also lead to a patient's energy demands being higher than usual. Protein is also lost in wound exudate.

If a patient is unable to maintain a good nutritional status, dietary supplements may be necessary, in the form of tablets (e.g. zinc supplements, multivitamins), by injection (e.g. Neocytamen, iron), or as food supplements or meal replacements.

Obese patients have reduced oxygen pressures in their tissues (Armstrong 1998). Adipose tissue is poorly networked by blood

Table 3.2 Important nutrients in wound healing

Nutrient	Role in healing
Protein	Repair and replacement of tissue
Carbohydrate	Energy, spares protein for wound healing
Vitamin C	Collagen synthesis, immunity
Vitamin B12	Protein synthesis
Zinc	Tissue repair, protein synthesis
Iron	Haemoglobin production
Copper	Increases the tensile strength of collagen

vessels so there are large areas of 'dead space' which reduce the oxygen tension. Production of collagen is also reduced and thus healing delayed (see Q1.8). Obesity is also a major risk factor in postoperative wound infection and the obese patient is more likely to suffer haematoma formation after surgery, which may delay healing by further reducing tissue oxygenation (Armstrong 1998).

For the patient with venous ulcers, the control of obesity is an important factor in ulcer healing, reducing prolonged back pressure in the venous system caused by deep vein obstruction in the pelvic area. Reducing obesity will also facilitate increased mobility and reduce venous stasis (see Q8.14 and Q8.28).

When discussing issues such as weight control and diet, it is important to be sure of the patient's level of understanding. This is illustrated in the following two scenarios.

Case study 2

Nurse A was asked to visit Miss P. An assessment indicated that she had a venous ulcer. Miss P was 43 years old, moderately overweight and had slight learning difficulties. Her mobility was impaired by both her weight and swelling in her legs. Nurse A instigated a treatment regimen of an alginate dressing and single-layer compression. She also gave advice about elevating the legs when sitting, trying some moderate exercise and losing weight.

Over the next few weeks, the ulcer decreased in size and the oedema was settling; Miss P had bought a large beanbag on which to elevate her legs, and had noticeably lost weight as her clothes appeared looser.

Nurse A did not see Miss P for several weeks as other staff undertook her care. When she went to reassess Miss P, the ulcer had almost healed, there was no oedema and an improvement in mobility was noted. Her weight appeared to have reduced considerably over a relatively short period. When nurse A instigated a discussion about diet, it became apparent that Miss P had cut out virtually all food except fruit and vegetables. She explained that dinner that day had been a bowl of broccoli. She knew these foods were good for her – the nurse had said plenty of fruit and vegetables – but she had no concept of her body's need for protein and some fat and carbohydrate. Nurse A had assumed this level of understanding. After a detailed discussion a more healthy diet with a slower level of weight loss was established.

Case study 3

Mrs R was an extremely obese woman of 38. Her weight was estimated to be in excess of 40 stones but an accurate measurement was difficult to obtain. She had an extensively ulcerated leg, which failed to respond to treatment, and was difficult to dress or bandage because of the shape of the limb. She was basically confined to the downstairs of the house because of her obesity. She had been previously advised to lose weight and had been seen by a dietitian to no effect.

On a joint visit between the district nurse and GP, Mrs R was told that if her weight did not reduce she stood no chance of her wounds healing, and she was endangering her life. Mrs R agreed to try to stick to a low-fat diet.

Several weeks later there appeared to be no change in her size and she was getting despondent. Both she and her husband were adamant that she was sticking to a low-fat diet.

The nurse decided to try to probe a bit deeper into exactly what Mrs R was eating. It transpired that most food was prepackaged and labelled low or lower fat. This included cheese, cream, crisps and chips. But lower fat than what? Again detailed discussion about food shattered the myths and enabled Mrs R to make a more successful attempt at weight loss.

> Q3.5 What dietary advice should be given to help improve wound healing in a poorly nourished patient?

- Encourage a high energy intake, such as sandwiches, cakes, biscuits and chocolate.

- Encourage a high protein intake, such as meat, fish, poultry, eggs and dairy foods.
- Encourage small but frequent snacks.
- Ensure that any supplements prescribed are palatable and sip feeds are the right flavour and temperature.
- Take care with foods that have low energy density such as fruit and vegetables. They contain essential micronutrients but the patient may feel full before their energy needs are met (Guest and Pearson 1997).

Q3.6   What should be included in a nutritional assessment?

The patient's history is important. This should include the following:

- What is the patient's normal diet?
- Have there been any recent changes or unintentional weight loss? Observe if the patient's clothes fit.
- Physical measurements such as weight and height will allow calculation of the body mass index.
- Direct observation of muscle bulk, subcutaneous fat, dehydrated skin and the patient's grip strength will aid assessment.
- A nutritional assessment scale may be useful, along with fluid balance and food intake charts if appropriate.

If necessary, involve the community dietitian. The patient should be regularly reassessed by weighing and monitoring intake. This should all be recorded on the care plan to allow evaluation.

Q3.7   Are supplements of vitamins and zinc useful to promote wound healing?

The recommended intake of vitamin C for a healthy adult is 40 mg/day (Department of Health 1991). The sick may require more, but how much more is uncertain. It is suggested that patients with pressure ulcers should always be suspected of being deficient as a result of factors such as chronic serious illness and institutionalised diets (Dickerson 1993). The best way to reach the requirement is by dietary intake, but if the patient is suspected to be deficient it is usual to give up to 1000 mg/day split into four doses. Higher doses should be avoided because of a relatively low renal threshold (Dickerson 1993).

Zinc deficiency may be prevalent in individuals with chronic malnutrition and will lead to difficulties with wound healing, and the liability of wound dehiscence and wound infection (Dickerson 1993). Supplementation is usually 660 mg/day split into three doses, but may carry the risk of copper depletion (Lewis 1998). There is no point in supplements if the patient is not depleted.

If a wound is failing to heal and zinc deficiency is suspected, a blood test may be taken. For further information on nutrition, the reader is referred to Buttriss, Wynne and Stanner, *Nutrition: A Handbook for Community Nurses* – in this series.

Q3.8   What drug therapy affects wound healing?

Drugs taken therapeutically for other conditions may inhibit wound healing (see Q6.2), including:

- Anti-inflammatory drugs, both steroidal and non-steroidal, will delay wound healing. These are commonly used to treat arthritis, which is often a problem in elderly people.
- Aspirin, commonly self-administered or given to treat circulatory disease, will also delay healing. These drugs are designed to suppress inflammation, which is essential for tissue repair (see Q1.8).
- Immunosuppressive drugs inhibit white cell activity and so delay the clearance of wound debris. Patients on these drugs are at high risk of developing a wound infection and may require prophylactic antimicrobial therapy and careful monitoring. Thought needs to be given to timing appointments for these patients to reduce the risks of cross-infection, such as before seeing any other patients who may have an infected wound.
- Cytotoxic drugs arrest cell division and also reduce protein production. This is true for both malignant cells and those vital for tissue repair.

Q3.9   How does smoking affect wound healing?

Smoking alters platelet function with a higher risk of clots blocking smaller vessels. Smokers also have reduced haemoglobin function (David 1986). This means less haemoglobin is available for oxygen transport, thus adversely affecting wound healing. The risk of arterial disease is also increased which may cause ischaemia and necrosis (see Q8.15).

Q3.10 How does alcohol affect wound healing?

Patients who are heavy drinkers may have liver disease. This may result in a reduction in the number of platelets and in clotting function. They may also have a lower resistance to infection. Gastritis and diarrhoea may predispose to malnourishment through malabsorption and anaemia caused by blood loss.

Q3.11 Do social factors have a role in wound healing?

Research suggests that there is a strong link between a person's social circumstances and his or her health (Miller 1999). The Black Report (Black 1982) found that people in the lower socioeconomic groups experienced poorer health and earlier death than those in the higher groups. Patients from these groups may be more likely to eat a less nutritious diet or to smoke cigarettes which will impair wound healing.

Psychological factors also play a part in wound healing. Experience shows that, if a patient develops venous leg ulcers, and previous generations in their family had had ulcers that failed to heal, their expectations of a positive outcome are lower and they may be less willing to tolerate treatments, such as compression bandaging, because they view them as pointless. Other patients are often suspected of tampering with their dressings and scratching the affected area, causing tissue damage. This may be because they fail to understand the importance of this or because they like to see the nurse and would rather their wound failed to heal.

Summary

If the chosen topical treatment is not having the desired effect, consider the other factors that may be impeding wound healing. The patient's age, concurrent disease(s) and general lifestyle factors are all pertinent for wound healing. Give the patient clear lifestyle advice, check that he or she understands that advice and reinforce it when appropriate.

CHAPTER 4

Wound cleansing

The topic of wound cleansing has often been surrounded with controversy. To clean or not to clean? This chapter discusses what constitutes best practice when cleansing a wound, what solutions are appropriate and when wound cleansing is necessary. The following information is pertinent for community nurses, although it may not be applicable to all hospital departments.

Q4.1   Why should cotton wool not be used to clean wounds?

It is generally accepted that cleansing wounds by swabbing with cotton wool or gauze results in the materials shedding fibres into the wound, which may act as a focus for infection (Draper 1985). Despite this, dressing packs available on the drug tariff all contain cotton-wool balls; these should be discarded. Vigorous swabbing may also damage healthy tissue. Gentle irrigation is therefore generally the preferred method.

Q4.2   When should wounds be cleansed?

Which wounds will benefit from cleansing? Traumatic wounds that contain particles of dirt or other matter will benefit from vigorous irrigation (Lawrence 1997). Wounds may also benefit from cleansing to remove gross exudate, remains of previous topical applications or crusting (Miller and Dyson 1996; Lawrence 1997). Bacteria are not removed but merely redistributed around the wound surface. It is pointless to cleanse wounds routinely; it is appropriate only to remove debris or old dressing material.

Reasons for not cleansing should be explained to the patient to avoid any misunderstandings, because most patients think that cleansing is essential.

Q4.3   What fluids are recommended for cleansing wounds, as I've been told antiseptics are of little value?

The most frequently used fluids are tap water, physiological ('normal') saline or antiseptics.

There is little evidence to suggest that use of antiseptics reduces the bacterial content of wounds. Wounds do not need to be sterile to heal. Current thinking suggests that the use of antiseptics is not advantageous in optimising wound healing. Some of the criticisms against antiseptics are listed in Box 4.1.

Preferred wound cleansing agents are described in Box 4.2. The safer antiseptic options are suggested by Lawrence (1997).

Box 4.1 Disadvantages of antiseptics in wound healing

Antiseptics do not come into contact with bacteria for long enough to kill them during normal wound cleansing

Bacteria may become resistant to antiseptics and those antiseptics containing cetrimide or chlorhexidine under certain conditions

The frequent use of antiseptics may contribute towards bacterial resistance to antibiotics (no link proven as yet)

Antiseptics adversely affect blood flow in the healing wound

Organic matter such as pus and wound exudate inactivates antiseptics

(Miller and Dyson 1996)

Q4.4   How can physiological saline be warmed before use?

The simplest way to warm saline before wound cleansing is to place the sachet, pod or canister in a suitable container such as a jug, mug or kidney dish that has warm water in it. This will raise the temperature without any risk of contamination The solution should be at body temperature when used.

Q4.5   What is an emollient?

Emollients are designed either as creams or for adding to baths/buckets of water to soothe and rehydrate dry scaled areas of

---

Box 4.2 Preferred wound cleansing agents

Chlorhexidine solutions: this is a good skin and hard surface disinfectant and shows
  low toxicity to living tissue in animal models (see Q10.9)
Povidone–iodine: iodine kills bacteria rapidly, possibly within a few seconds, but can
  impair the microcirculation in animals
Tap water: one study conducted with tap water found that there were fewer infections
  in wounds cleansed with tap water and that no bacteria were transferred to the
  wound (Angeras et al. 1991). However, some cell damage may occur as a result of
  osmotic pressure and this may cause pain (Lawrence 1997). Leg ulcers may be
  cleansed in a bucket of warm water (see Q8.25)
Saline in a 0.9% (physiological) solution: has similar osmotic pressures to the tissue in
  mammals. This reinforces the fact that saline baths are inappropriate because the
  concentrations vary widely. Saline is currently favoured as the treatment of choice,
  minimising the risk of tissue damage and pain. This should be used as a warm solution (see Q5.3)

---

skin. If used in water it does not matter if they touch the ulcer itself
(see Q8.25).

Summary

Wounds should be gently irrigated and not swabbed. Clean wounds
only if it is necessary to remove debris such as the remains of dressings or exudate. Warm saline is the preferred cleansing lotion.

CHAPTER 5

Dressings

Many types of wound dressings are now available and it can be diffi-cult to choose the one most appropriate to the wound. This chapter attempts to place the dressings into broad categories with some suggestions for their appropriate use. The dressings mentioned are not the only ones available and for further information it would be appropriate to refer to a text such as the *Formulary of Wound Manage-ment Products* (Morgan 1994). Your primary care group, or trust, may have a wound care formulary that recommends specific products.

For information about methods of application, time between dressing changes, removal and contraindications, see the manufac-turers' instructions. Only dressings on the drug tariff are discussed.

It is important that the chosen dressing is appropriate to the wound, that it has been proved to be clinically effective and that it is cost-effective. This chapter looks at some of the products available and in what circumstances they may be beneficial although, as new products are becoming available constantly, it is inevitable that some recent developments are not covered. Dealing with allergic reactions is also discussed.

Q5.1 Ideally a wound should have a moist healing environment. How is this achieved in practice?

A primary factor in optimising healing is that the dressing should provide a moist environment (see Q1.9). All modern occlusive dress-ings should provide this type of environment. No dry dressings should be used on open wounds because these will allow the area to dry out and thus impede healing (see Q5.5).

One notable exception to this is in the case of peripheral necrosis secondary to arterial disease (e.g. necrotic toes, peripheral diabetic ulcers) where moisture may increase the risk of rapid infection (see Q8.20).

Q5.2   How can maceration from exudate be avoided?

The wound should be kept free from excessive exudate. Although the wound needs to be kept moist, it must not be wet. This will allow the skin to become soggy and macerated and may lead to further tissue breakdown. A dressing should be selected that provides the correct absorbency and the frequency of dressing changes should reflect the anticipated level of exudate. All dressings are designed with particular types of wounds in mind, e.g. alginates are designed for highly exuding wounds (see Q5.9) and vapour-permeable films for wounds with very little exudate (see Q5.18). This is an important criterion in dressing selection (see also Q11.5).

Q5.3   Does temperature have an effect on wound healing?

Wound healing is optimised when wounds are kept at body temperature. If the temperature of the wound drops, mitotic activity slows down thus reducing wound healing. A drop in wound temperature also disrupts leukocytic activity and oxyhaemoglobin dissociation (Thomas 1990; Miller and Dyson 1996).

Lock (1980) and Myers (1982) found that after cleansing it could take a wound up to 40 minutes to regain body temperature and a further 3 hours for mitotic activity to return to normal. Thus it is advisable to warm saline before wound cleansing (see Q4.4), to keep wounds exposed for as short a time as possible, to try not to disturb wounds unnecessarily and to consider the type of material being used, i.e. cotton gauze will keep a wound at around 27°C whereas a hydrocolloid or foam dressing will increase the temperature to 35°C (Thomas 1990).

Q5.4   Can micro-organisms get under dressings?

The dressing should be impermeable to micro-organisms. This should work both ways. While micro-organisms should be kept away from wounds, it is also undesirable to have micro-organisms from a wound spreading to the environment.

Any non-adhesive dressing should be taped like a 'picture frame' if the surrounding skin is in good condition, or bandaged to cover the dressing completely.

If 'strike-through' (exudate seeps through or under the edges of the dressing) occurs, a warm wet passage is created for micro-organisms. Secondary padding should be applied or the wound redressed (see Q5.23). The patient should be advised that, if leakage occurs, he or she should cover it with a dressing pad while awaiting a district nurse visit or surgery appointment.

Q5.5   Can I use traditional gauze as a primary dressing?

Dressings should not shed particles on to a wound. Modern dressings are designed to high standards and will not shed fibres on to the wound surface. However, traditional gauze, lint or cotton wool all shed fibres which can serve as a focus for infection.

In addition, the dressing should not cause trauma to the wound. If the chosen dressing adheres to the wound, trauma and pain may occur when the dressing is removed (see Q2.7). The ideal healing environment should be free from materials that adhere; this is provided by all modern dressings.

For both of these reasons, traditional dressings such as cotton gauze and paraffin gauze should not be used on open wounds. Adherence occurs as the wound exudate becomes incorporated into the gauze and dries out, adhering to the tissue below. Removal causes the top layer of granulation tissue to be removed with the dressing. Paraffin gauze leaves a criss-cross pattern where new granulation tissue has grown through the mesh, illustrating this quite graphically.

Q5.6   Are occlusive dressings recommended?

Occlusive dressings stop any atmospheric oxygen getting to the wound. It has been noted that angiogenesis (formation of new blood vessels) in granulating wounds takes place rapidly in the hypoxic environment of occlusive dressings such as hydrocolloids (Cherry and Ryan 1985). However, when a wound begins to show signs of new epidermis forming, it appears to happen more rapidly in a more oxygen-rich environment (Silver 1985). It may be appropriate to use an occlusive dressing when a wound needs to granulate, but to switch to an oxygen-permeable dressing (e.g. a foam dressing) to encourage epithelialisation (see Q1.8 and Q2.13).

Q5.7   Some dressings are not available on prescription. Can they still be used?

Many nurses have arrangements where they order one item from a pharmacist and exchange it for another product of the same value. This is illegal! Even though it is done with the patient's best interests at heart, this action constitutes fraud. If prosecuted the nurse could face a fine, imprisonment and dismissal.

Q5.8   What factors should be considered when choosing a dressing?

Here is a list of areas to consider. The dressing should have the following qualities:

- Safe to use, i.e. has been proved safe and effective by clinical trials
- Acceptable to the patient
- Cost-effective; do not just think in terms of unit cost
- Capable of standardisation and evaluation
- Allows monitoring of the wound
- Provides mechanical protection
- Non-flammable
- Sterilisable
- Comfortable and mouldable
- Requires infrequent changing.

Currently, no one dressing meets all these criteria. Therefore it is important to assess the wound thoroughly, decide on a treatment goal and select the most appropriate dressing from those available.

If the wound does not respond to the chosen dressing, it is important to remember that the dressing plays only a part in the healing process and any underlying causes must be treated and factors affecting healing reviewed (see Q3.1–Q3.7).

Q5.9   What is an alginate dressing?

These dressings are made from seaweed, which contains large quantities of alginate. They are highly absorbent so they should not be used on wounds with very little exudate, because they will adhere to the wound surface. Some clinicians wet the dressing with saline, but this seems pointless as the dressing is designed to be highly absorbent and, on a dry wound, will dry out at body temperature. All alginates are highly absorbent and form a gel on contact with wound exudate, giving a moist environment while absorbing excess fluid. They may be used on flat wounds and also to pack cavity wounds. Some are manufactured as ropes and ribbons especially for packing. They also have haemostatic qualities and so are excellent for managing some minor surgical bleeds and minor injuries (see Q6.6 and Q7.11). A secondary dressing is required (see Q5.23). Examples of alginates are Kaltostat (Convatec), SeaSorb (Coloplast), Sorbsan and Sorbsan Plus (Pharma-Plast, Tegagen (3M), Algosteril (Biersdorf), Algisite Plus (Smith & Nephew) and Melgisorb (Monlycke).

Q5.10 What are bead dressings?

These dressings are made up of polysaccharide beads. They are indicated for wet sloughy wounds and should not be used on clean or dry wounds. The beads are extremely hydrophilic and will cause pain if the wound is too dry (see Q2.7). The ones in most common usage are Iodosorb and Iodoflex (Smith & Nephew). Both contain iodine and have been used with some success on wounds with superficial infection or superficial wounds contaminated with methicillin-resistant *Staphylococcus aureus* (MRSA) (see Q10.7 and Q10.13). All require a secondary dressing (see Q5.23).

Q5.11 What is an enzyme dressing?

Varidase (Wyath Labs) is a dry powder containing two enzymes, streptokinase and streptodornase. Varidase is designed to débride necrotic or very sloughy wounds (see Q2.10 and Q2.11). The powder can be reconstituted with sterile saline and applied to dry scabs that have been cross-hatched with a scalpel as a soak. Some practitioners do inject under scabs, but this must be done with care so that healthy tissue is not affected and this method is not generally recommended. An alternative is to reconstitute the powder with 5 ml sterile water and mix with 15 ml intrasite gel. Whichever method of application is chosen, a secondary dressing is required.

When mixing Varidase powder with any solution, care must be taken not to shake the vial vigorously or the enzymes will become denatured and the treatment ineffective.

Q5.12 Can the use of topical streptokinase affect the treatment of myocardial infarction?

All patients treated with Varidase show an increase in antistreptokinase titres. Morgan (1994) recommends that it would be sensible not to use it on patients at risk of myocardial infarction.

Bux et al. (1997) conducted a study to assess antistreptokinase levels in patients treated with intravenous streptokinase for acute myocardial infarction, and in patients treated with topical streptokinase for cutaneous wounds. He found that topical application of streptokinase causes a significant humoral response for 1 month which then declines over a 6-month period. This antibody response is significantly lower than when streptokinase is given intravenously. Bux et al. conclude that, if a patient has been treated with topical streptokinase in the last 6 months, it would be prudent to avoid intravenous streptokinase and an alternative thrombolytic should be used in the treatment of a myocardial infarction.

Another small study by Green (1993) measured the antistreptokinase titres of five patients treated with topical Varidase, who all showed an increased titre. He concluded that the use of Varidase should be restricted to those not at risk of a myocardial infarction.

Q5.13 What are foam dressings?

Foam dressings (including hydropolymer and hydrocellular dressings) are generally highly absorbent and create a moist environment for wound healing. They can be used on a wide variety of wounds although, if the wound is very dry, they may stick.

These dressings are available without adhesive, which is useful if the surrounding skin is fragile or damaged, or as adhesive dressings. They can be used on their own or as a secondary dressing, e.g. with hydrogels (see Q5.23).

Some non-adhesive foams include Allevyn (Smith & Nephew), Lyofoam and Lyofoam Extra (Seton). Lyofoam is useful for resolving overgranulation.

Adhesive foams include Allevyn Adhesive (Smith & Nephew), CombiDERM (Convatec) and Tielle (Johnson & Johnson).

Q5.14 What are hydrofibre dressings?

Hydrofibre dressings are made of 100% sodium carboxymethylcellulose. This is the main ingredient of hydrocolloid dressings and it is spun into fibres and made into sheets or ribbon dressings. It absorbs fluid directly into its fibre structure. In the presence of exudate it converts into a soft gel sheet which maintains a warm, moist, local wound condition.

Hydrofibre dressings will absorb moderate-to-large quantities of exudate, locking it away from good skin and preventing maceration. They can be used to treat a variety of wounds, sloughy or clean, flat or cavities (Williams 1999). They are used for wounds similar to those dressed by alginates. They always require a secondary dressing (see Q5.23).

An example of a hydrofibre dressing is Aquacel (Convatec).

Q5.15 What are hydrogels?

Amorphous hydrogels have a high water content. They are very useful for débriding or desloughing wounds by rehydrating the dead tissue, thus allowing the body to shed this tissue by autolysis. Gels are designed to be used on flat wounds and to fill cavities. They are also reported to reduce pain at the wound site (Morgan 1994). They require a secondary dressing (see Q5.23).

Examples of hydrogels are Intrasite Gel (Smith & Nephew), Nu-Gel (Johnson & Johnson), Sterigel (Seton) and Purilon Gel (Coloplast).

Q5.16 What are hydrocolloids?

Hydrocolloid dressings are made from combinations of synthetic polymers and are one of the oldest of the 'modern' dressings; they are used in many situations. These dressings are waterproof, adhesive and interactive, and form a gel on contact with wound exudate. This may have a slight odour, which is normal, and it is advisable to warn the patient so that he or she does not get upset if this occurs.

Hydrocolloids can aid desloughing (see Q2.11) and can be used on wounds with light-to-medium exudate. Their occlusive nature gives a hypoxic environment, which stimulates angiogenesis (see Q5.6), and the moist environment gives pain relief by keeping nerve endings moist (see Q1.9). Examples of hydrocolloids are Comfeel (Coloplast), Granuflex (Convatec) and Tegasorb (3M).

Extra thin versions are also available: Comfeel Transparent (Coloplast) and Duoderm (Convatec).

All hydrocolloids can be used alone or as a secondary dressing (check manufacturers' recommendations) (see Q5.23).

Q5.17 What is a hydrocolloid gel dressing?

Granugel (Convatec) is a gel that contains hydrocolloid for desloughing and débriding wounds (see Q2.10 and Q2.11) and can also be applied to clean wounds. It requires a secondary dressing such as Granuflex (see Q5.16).

Q5.18 What are vapour-permeable film dressings?

These were the first modern dressings to be produced. Waterproof adhesive films create a moist environment but have no fluid-handling capabilities. They can be used on superficial wounds with minimal exudate, prophylactically, e.g. to reduce shearing forces, on wounds healing by primary intention or as a secondary dressing securing other products (see Q5.23). They have the advantage of allowing the wound to be observed for any adverse happenings such as infection, e.g. over a suture line (see Q6.1). Examples of film dressings are Bioclusive (Johnson & Johnson), Opsite Flexigrid (Smith & Nephew), Tegaderm (3M), Cutifilm (Biersdorf) and Mefilm (Monlycke).

Q5.19 Can proflavine cream be used to pack wounds?

Proflavine cream is an antimicrobial preparation of doubtful efficacy, which was popular at one time for packing a wound such as pilonidal sinus (see Q6.3). It is mildly bacteriostatic against some Gram-positive bacteria, but less effective against Gram-negative organisms such as *Proteus* and *Pseudomonas* spp. and *Escherichia coli*.

If the cream is a water-in-oil emulsion, the proflavine has very little antibacterial activity because it is not released from the emulsion base.

Hypersensitivity has been reported because the cream contains lanolin, a known sensitising agent (see Q5.20).

Q5.20   What common irritants and allergens likely to cause contact dermatitis may be found in wound care products?

Lanolin

Lanolin (wool alcohol) is a known sensitiser. It can be found in many creams, ointments, bath additives, baby products and barrier preparations. It is better not to use any products containing lanolin on the skin around leg ulcers.

Antibiotics

Neomycin and framycetin are topical antibiotics that are commonly reported as skin sensitisers. When managing leg ulcers, gentamicin and bacitracin are also significant sensitisers (Cameron 1998). Topical antibiotics are found in creams, ointments, tulle dressings and medicated powders. They are best avoided because of the problems of both sensitisation and resistant bacteria.

Alcohol

Cetyl alcohol, stearyl alcohol and cetylstearyl alcohol are emulsifiers. These are difficult to avoid because they are found in many popular leg ulcer preparations such as aqueous creams, corticosteroid creams, moisturisers, some paste bandages and emulsifying ointments.

Rubber

Rubber may be found in elastic bandages, some support hosiery, tubular elastic supports and latex gloves. If the patient has a rubber allergy, the nurse should wear vinyl gloves.

Parabens

The parabens group of preservatives possess antibacterial and antifungal properties; they are widely used preservatives in topical medicaments, moisturisers and some paste bandages.

Ester of resin

Colophony (an ester of resin) is found in the adhesive backing of some plasters, tapes and dressings.

Fragrances

Fragrances used in many over-the-counter products such as bath additives and moisturisers may cause sensitisation.

> Q5.21 How can irritants and allergens best be avoided?

The following measures can be taken to minimise the risk of contact dermatitis, particularly if the patient is known to be sensitive to a variety of preparations:

- Use warm physiological saline (0.9%) to irrigate leg ulcers or wash the leg with plain warm tap water (see Q4.3, Q4.4, Q5.3 and Q8.25).
- Avoid using topical antibiotics or antiseptics (see Q4.3).
- Do not use adhesive tape directly on to the skin.
- Use a simple emollient such as 50% white soft paraffin, 50% liquid paraffin; this can be made up by the pharmacist.
- Do not use any product containing lanolin (see Q5.20).
- Avoid creams; use ointments instead.
- Do not apply elastic bandages directly on to the skin.
- Wear vinyl not latex gloves.
- Discourage the patient from using over-the-counter preparations for self-treatment.
- Consider referring the patient to a dermatologist for patch testing if the patient is known to be sensitive to a range of products.

> Q5.22 Can wound dressings be combined?

Many combinations are frequently seen, but far less research about the clinical effectiveness of such treatments is available. Manufacturers of dressings do not normally make statements about their dressings in combination with other products because the range of primary and secondary dressings is vast. If manufacturers happen to make examples of both product types, they may well be prepared to provide some assurances that their products used in combination are safe (Thomas and Vowden 1998). If in doubt about the safety of a combination, a company helpline or a pharmacist may be able to answer your query.

Also remember that, if a skin reaction occurs, you may not be able to tell which of the products has caused it, which may limit future management.

Q5.23 What types of dressings can be used as secondary dressings?

Low adherence dressings such as N-A Dressing or Tricotex can be used over gels, creams, alginates, etc. These are simple dressings with no absorbency and may need more substantial padding over them.

Padding such as Gamgee products should be used only over a suitable primary dressing that protects the wound from any loose fibres, which may become incorporated into the wound causing adherence. Placed over a suitable dressing, it does allow easy passage of fluid.

More modern pads such as the Surgipad are available; these are sleeved to prevent loose fibres entering the wound and for this reason should not be cut. Unless strike-through occurs they give a reasonable barrier to bacteria (Thomas 1998) (see Q5.4).

Orthopaedic wadding, which was originally designed for use under plaster casts, is now frequently used under compression bandaging both to protect bony prominences and to absorb exudate (see Q8.29).

Vapour-permeable film dressings, designed as a primary dressing for superficial low exudate wounds, can also be used to prevent moisture loss from hydrogels applied to dry wounds or wounds with low exudate (see Q5.18). They may also be used over alginates.

There is a growing trend to use hydrocolloid dressings over gels and alginates. Although this may be acceptable in some instances, it should be remembered that some hydrocolloids can absorb a considerable amount of fluid and may therefore reduce a hydrogel's ability to rehydrate a wound. The clinical significance of this has not been determined (Thomas 1998).

Foam dressings are usually used alone but, as with hydrocolloids, there is a trend to use them in combination with gels and alginates (see Q5.13). There is no published evidence to support this practice and again they may take up moisture from a gel, but this does not seem to occur to any great extent and slightly more gel could be applied to stop this effect (Stevens 1998). A gel/foam combination may then be a benefit if the wound is producing a high level of exudate, but for dry necrotic or sloughy wounds it is difficult to justify the cost (Thomas 1998).

If a wound is malodorous, dressings containing activated charcoal may be appropriate (see Q2.6). These fit into two categories: those intended as primary dressings such as Actisorb Plus, Lyofoam C and Carboflex, and those intended as secondary dressings such as Clini-Sorb or Denidor. Although they have no odour-absorbing properties, occlusive products such as film dressings or hydrocolloids may reduce odour by preventing the escape of volatile molecules that are responsible for the smell (Thomas 1998).

Q5.24 Are there any products that should be avoided with vegetarian patients?

Most products are suitable, although some hydrocolloids may contain gelatin, which is an animal derivative, whereas other dressings may not. Fibracol is a collagen alginate that contains over 90% bovine collagen, so it is unsuitable for a vegetarian patient.

If necessary check with the product manufacturer.

Summary

No one dressing will meet all the criteria for the ideal wound dressing. Traditional dressings such as gauze should not be used as a primary dressing on any open wounds. The chosen dressing should be the one most suited to the stage of healing, exudate level and patient satisfaction. Avoid irritants and allergens; document any known allergies for future reference. If combining dressings, consider whether they are likely to counteract each other or react with each other and whether the combination is cost-effective.

CHAPTER 6

Surgical wounds

Community nurses are often asked to manage postoperative surgical wounds following early patient discharge from hospital. Many GPs undertake minor surgery within the practice; this is expected to rise under the changing health care initiatives.

This chapter examines management of surgical wounds, and considers factors that may affect healing which are particular to these wounds. Pilonidal sinuses and abscesses are also discussed in the following text as these are frequently managed within the community setting.

Q6.1   How should surgical wounds be managed?

Surgical wounds are usually closed with sutures or clips, which are left in place for 5–7 days depending on the type of surgery, and the depth of the wound they are closing (see Q1.6)

Studies have shown that after 24 hours the skin will have formed a natural barrier at the suture or clip line which means a dressing may be unnecessary (Chrintz 1989). Patients will require dressings if there is any leakage from the suture line or to protect the wound from rubbing on clothing. Some areas, such as the groin after varicose vein surgery, may be particularly prone to friction and may require a light dressing to absorb any perspiration and to reduce friction. As the skin edges have been brought together traditional dressings such as gauze or Melolin are often used. However, these may not be comfortable and are not waterproof (Miller 1995) (see Q5.5). It may be appropriate to consider a more modern alternative such as a vapour-permeable film (see Q5.18), a polyurethane dressing (see Q5.13) or a thin hydrocolloid (see Q5.16). Advantages of these dressings include comfort and less bulk, they do not require bandaging or taping into position, are waterproof and in most cases can be left in position until the sutures or clips can be removed. (Thomas 1990). Once sutures or clips have been removed, a dressing should not be necessary unless the wound continues to exude from any areas along the suture line.

Advice given to the patient may include covering the wound for 24 hours after surgery. If the wound then appears dry, he or she may shower, but should avoid bathing because this will reduce the natural barrier. While awaiting the removal of sutures or clips, the patient should observe the wound for any signs of infection (see Q10.1) and seek medical aid if any of these occur.

Q6.2   What factors can affect the healing of surgical wounds?

The patient's physiological condition and the surgical and nursing environment will have a profound effect on wound healing. As with all wounds factors such as ageing, underlying disease, nutrition and lifestyle will affect healing (see Q3.2–Q3.11).

The length of hospital stay before surgery has been suggested as a factor affecting postoperative recovery (Partridge 1998). Trauma patients requiring surgery or those with a preoperative illness appear to heal more slowly.

Other concurrent therapies may also delay healing (see Q3.9). Corticosteroids will affect all stages of healing. Immunosuppressive drugs delay the inflammatory response in wound healing, which results in a reduced white blood cell count, increasing susceptibility to infection (David 1986). Anticoagulants are sometimes given prophylactically when patients have major surgery. These impair blood clotting and may result in haematoma formation. Cytotoxic drugs interfere with cell replication by suppressing the inflammatory response and protein synthesis in patients who are already debilitated from a malignant disease (Bland et al. 1984). Radiotherapy can also damage skin by decreasing vascularity and fibrosis (Cutting and Harding 1994), which makes it more vulnerable to trauma as well as reducing the patient's non-specific cell-mediated response to bacterial invasion. Penicillin interferes with collagen formation and will decrease a wound's tensile strength (Cooper 1990) (see Q1.8).

Wound infection can also be a complication of wound healing (see Q10.1 and Q10.2). Infection rates are higher in patients who are old, obese, taking steroids, malnourished or diabetic, and those with longer preoperative stays (Partridge 1998).

Patients who are undergoing surgery may also suffer stress and anxiety. Although the relationship to wound healing is not fully understood this appears to impair the healing process. Stress and anxiety may also reduce motivation and interfere with rest and sleep which is important to optimise wound healing.

Q6.3   What is a pilonidal sinus?

The most common site for a pilonidal sinus is between the buttocks in the upper natal cleft. It is generally accepted that it is an acquired abnormality (Gould 1997; Hodgkin 1998).

Pilonidal disease starts at the onset of puberty when the sex hormones begin to affect sebaceous glands in the natal cleft. A hair follicle becomes distended with keratin to form an asymptomatic cyst. Gradually a combination of friction and trauma provoke an inflammatory response (see Q1.8).

Patients may present with a pilonidal abscess, with a short history of intense pain, swelling and redness around the infected area. Alternatively, they may have moderate-to-mild pain and a history of recurrent discharge.

Patients are usually between the age of puberty up to 40 years. Men are twice as likely as women to develop this disease, presumably because they are more hirsute (Gould 1997).

Q6.4   What is the recommended treatment for pilonidal disease?

If an abscess has formed, it is treated as a surgical emergency and will require incision and drainage. The wound will require loose packing until it heals. Commonly used dressings are alginates or in some circumstances hydrogels (Gould 1997) (see Q5.9 and Q5.15). Traditionally, ribbon gauze soaked in a solution such as proflavine (see Q5.19) was used, but this is no longer recommended. Gauze may dry out and cause trauma and pain on removal and may also shed fibres into the wound, so it should not be used (see Q5.5).

If no abscess has formed there are several options, although treatment is controversial (Hodgkin 1998). Hair can be removed with forceps and curette, if the sinus is small and not infected. The patient can have phenol injections as an outpatient, or surgical treatments include laying the area open to permit drainage and allow healing by secondary intention (see Q1.7). On occasion the area can be opened and hairs and debris removed, followed by primary closure.

Q6.5   What is an abscess and how should incision and drainage be managed?

An abscess is a localised collection of pus, comprising exudate, bacteria, dead white cells and the partial liquefaction of other cells and tissue. The infection becomes walled off by granulation tissue and a layer of dead white cells. As the abscess increases in size, the internal pressure increases and this produces pain.

The usual treatment is surgical incision of the abscess and drainage of the contents (The Wound Programme 1992). The resulting cavity is then packed with a dressing such as an alginate or hydrofibre dressing (Q5.9 and Q5.14), which allows for future drainage. Antibiotics penetrate poorly into an abscess but serve as an adjunct to surgery.

Q6.6   Is there a recommended management following removal of ingrowing toenails?

The procedure for removal of part or all of an ingrowing toenail varies with the practitioner. Some doctors treat the area with phenol to prevent regrowth, others do not. Invariably the nail bed bleeds profusely. Use of a haemostatic dressing, such as an alginate (see Q5.9), covered with a foam dressing (see Q5.13) reduces adhesion of the dressing to the toe. The wound can be assessed after 3–4 days, when further management can be planned. The use of foam dressings on the feet appears to reduce pressure from footwear, which patients find comfortable. The use of tulle dressings is not recommended, because they adhere to the wound and cause damage on removal (see Q5.5).

Summary

Most surgical wounds are closed with the skin edges apposed and only a simple dressing is required. Several factors will affect the healing of surgical wounds, including length of hospital stay, poor health before surgery, concurrent therapies and wound infection. As with all wounds, the choice of dressing is directed by the individual wound state.

Chapter 7

Burns, scalds and minor injuries

The practice nurse is often consulted for advice and management of minor injuries, burns and scalds during the daily surgery. This chapter looks at the treatment of these conditions, because they are relevant to all community nurses. Recommendations are made as to which patients will require specialist advice. The aftercare of donor sites and management of scar tissue are also discussed. It is recognised that specialist centres may have their own regimen for the care of these wounds, and the reader is expected to follow local protocols.

> Q7.1 Patients with burns and scalds frequently attend the GP surgery. Which should be referred to accident and emergency?

As a general rule, patients fitting the following criteria should attend the accident and emergency department (Gower and Lawrence 1995):

- Any burn exceeding 5% of the body surface area.
- Burns of functionally important areas, such as the face, hands, feet, perineum, joints or flexor surfaces.
- If other injury is suspected, e.g. inhalation of smoke or other noxious gas or electric shock.
- Patients with diseases such as epilepsy or diabetes.
- If the burn will limit a person's ability to self-manage, e.g. to the hands of an elderly person living alone.
- Patients with full-thickness burns which may benefit from early grafting (see Figure 1.4).
- Anyone showing signs of local infection or evidence of septicaemia (see Tables 10.1 and 10.2).

- Burns that create doubt, such as non-accidental injury, or those of unknown depth, such as chemical or electrical burns.

Q7.2   How should sunburn be treated?

Frequently sunburn is erythema which will subside within 48 hours (Lawrence 1996), leaving no tissue damage. Cold water is effective for relieving the pain, while the usual treatment is reassurance and calamine lotion. If the skin has blistered, this is a sign of actual tissue loss. The burn should then be assessed to see whether it can be treated in the surgery or whether it will require hospital treatment. Patients attending with sunburn should be reminded of the potential dangers of sun damage in the development of skin cancer and advised on future protection.

Q7.3   What is the best treatment for minor burns and scalds?

If a patient in a nursing home suffers a minor burn or scald, or if a patient comes to the surgery immediately, the recommended first aid treatment for most burns is cold water for a minimum of 10 minutes or until the pain has decreased. This treatment is endorsed by the British Burns Association (Lawrence 1996). The purpose of this is to quench residual heat rapidly. Local cooling also has a marked analgesic effect. However, most patients will have suffered their burn or scald well in advance of attending the surgery.

Treatment will depend on the size, site and depth of the burn. If present, blisters should not be deroofed (Gower and Lawrence 1995). The absence of skin may allow for greater possibility of infection. If the blister is full of fluid and causing acute discomfort from pressure, aspiration under sterile conditions should be considered.

Very minor burns are often treated with simple tulle dressings. Those containing antibiotics should be avoided (see Q10.4). Silver sulphadiazine cream (Flamazine) is often applied under low adherent dressings or simple tulle, but may be difficult to secure and may cause maceration.

One suggested treatment regimen is:

- Day 1: Flamazine and tulle
- Day 2: tulle
- Day 5: tulle and review as necessary.

Other dressings that may be suitable include film dressings or hydrocolloid dressings (see Q5.16 and Q5.18). Most minor burns will heal within a week to 10 days; after this they should be dressed as appropriate. If the burn has not healed or almost healed within 3 weeks of injury, it may be full thickness and require a skin graft (Gower and Lawrence 1995) (see Figure 1.4).

Minor burns to the face where it is difficult to apply dressings may be treated with 10% aqueous povidone–iodine. This needs to be applied three to four times a day for 5–7 days. This will reduce the possibility of bacterial complications (see Box 4.2). Tetanus cover should also be reviewed.

Q7.4   Are there any instances when treatment for burns with cold water is not appropriate?

Cold water treatment is not appropriate if the burns have been caused by metallic sodium, potassium or calcium. These all react violently with any aqueous solution. These burns are rare and appropriate medical advice should be sought.

Q7.5   What advice should the patient be given when the burn has healed?

The new epithelium of a recently healed burn is delicate and sun sensitive. Dry dressings might initially be indicated for protection. Total sun block should be used if the area is exposed to sunlight and the area well moisturised with a simple non-perfumed cream.

If the burn was to the lower limb of an elderly patient, support bandages may be required to reduce the possibility of knocks to delicate skin resulting in episodes of ulceration (Gower and Lawrence 1995).

Q7.6   What advice should patients be given about caring for healed donor sites?

Most donor sites heal well with little scarring. The patient should be advised to protect the area from extremes of temperature, trauma and exposure to the sun (Fowler and Dempsey 1998). Skin should be moisturised with a simple non-perfumed cream to keep it supple and soft. If it is likely to be exposed to direct sunlight, a sun block of factor 25 or higher should be used.

Q7.7   What is a scar, and what advice can the patient be given for improving
        its appearance?

A scar is the mark left after a wound has healed. Damage to the
epidermis is healed by replacement of the epidermis and will
normally result only in slight scarring which will fade naturally. If
deeper tissue such as the dermis is damaged, the body lays down
collagen during the healing process (see Q1.8), and the resulting scar
will be much more noticeable. Often these do not fade and will
remain red or dark and raised. Scars can be described as hyper-
trophic, i.e. they remain in the original wound site and continue to
grow for up to 6 months, or they can be keloid – such scars grow
larger than the original wound and grow indefinitely.

A recently developed product, Circa-Care (Smith & Nephew), is
a sheet of silicone in an adhesive gel sheet. This is placed over the
scar for 2–4 months and has been shown to improve appearances in
90% of cases (data from Smith & Nephew). This product can be
bought from pharmacies, but is also available on FP10.

Q7.8   What is the preferred treatment for pretibial lacerations?

Pretibial lacerations often leave a flap of skin on the shin. Commonly
the patient has extremely fragile skin, so consideration is needed to
select a dressing that will not cause trauma from any adhesive on
removal. If the skin flap remains, it can be secured back into place
with adhesive strips (see Q7.9), but often the blood supply to the flap
is poor and the replaced flap will not remain viable.

Complications of pretibial lacerations include infection and/or
the deterioration of the wound into a chronic state (see Q8.1 and
Q8.32). If there are underlying problems with the venous circulation, a venous ulcer may result. Likewise, if the arterial circulation is
poor healing will be compromised (see Q3.9).

If the area of the laceration continues to ooze blood, an alginate
dressing such as Kaltostat may be used as a haemostat (see Q5.9).

Q7.9   When are adhesive wound closure strips appropriate?

Wound closure strips are appropriate for minor lacerations or minor
wounds where there is little force needed to keep the wound edges

together. They cause less trauma than sutures on both application and removal.

The following is the application procedure:

- Ensure that the surrounding skin is dry.
- Start by drawing the skin from each side of the wound together at the centre, ensuring that the strip adheres right up to the edge of the cut.
- More closures are then used to draw the sides of the wound together and gradually any gaps filled in to make a neat repair.
- A secondary dressing is placed over the closed wound (see Q5.23).

Once closed a small wound should have healed within 5–7 days (depending on position) and the strips may be removed.

Q7.10 When is surgical glue appropriate?

Surgical glue has been used in secondary care for many years. It is also a useful primary care tool. The use of surgical glue in primary care can reduce the need for suturing wounds, thus reducing the pain and anxiety in children. Surgical glue is particularly useful for closing small lacerations on the face and head, taking care to avoid the eye area. It is not recommended for body parts where tension occurs, e.g. the chin or on finger joints. Glue can be used in conjunction with adhesive strips.

Advantages of surgical glue include the following:

- Nurse-only management
- Speed of application
- No local anaesthetic required
- No follow-up for suture removal
- Reduced pain and anxiety, especially for children
- Reduced attendance at hospital.

The wound should be kept dry for 5 days. No follow-up is required unless the wound reopens. It can be reglued or sutured if appropriate.

Q7.11 Is there a simple method for managing lacerations?

Stanley knife blades are a common cause of lacerations, which often bleed profusely. Alginate dressings act as a haemostat, and if applied on to a bleeding wound which is then elevated the bleeding will reduce fairly quickly. It is essential to ensure that there is no foreign body in the wound before applying pressure; this is of particular relevance if the wound was caused by broken glass.

Summary

Only minor burns and scalds should be treated in the surgery; refer any of concern for secondary care management. In most instances, cold water is the most effective first aid measure. If patients attend with sunburn, consider health promotion issues; promote sunscreen and body protection to prevent further episodes of sunburn. Newly healed burns and donor sites should be protected from sunlight; high-factor sun lotion/sun block is recommended for these sites.

Adhesive strips and surgical glue are alternatives to suturing. Each has advantages and disadvantages, and these should be weighed against patient preference, cost-effectiveness and efficacy.

CHAPTER 8

Leg ulcers

The management of patients with leg ulcers is a problem commonly encountered by community nurses. Studies have shown that between 65% and 85% of patients are managed exclusively by the primary health care team (Kendrick et al. 1994). This care is costly. In 1990 Charing Cross Hospital leg ulcer service estimated the annual cost of treating a leg ulcer to be between £2700 and £5200 per patient. This suggests that the treatment of leg ulcers costs the National Health Service £300–600 million a year for the UK as a whole (Morison 1991).

Understanding the aetiology and management of both venous and arterial ulcers can reduce the morbidity of these conditions and improve the quality of life for patients.

Q8.1   What is a leg ulcer?

A leg ulcer can be defined as an area of discontinuity of the epidermis and dermis on the lower leg persisting for 4 weeks or more, excluding ulcers confined to the foot.

Q8.2   What are the principal causes of leg ulcers?

Leg ulcers may be caused by a number of underlying pathologies. Minor trauma is often the immediate cause of the ulcer but underlying pathology leads to ulcer development. The most common of these pathologies is venous disease (see Q8.14), which accounts for about 70% of ulcers. Around 10–15% are the result of arterial disease (see Q8.15). About 10% of patients will have both venous and arterial disease. These ulcers are known as mixed aetiology ulcers.

Q8.3   Are there any other causes of leg ulcers to consider?

Around 2–5% of patients develop ulcers as a result of other causes. Although rare these should be kept in mind. Some of these are listed in Table 8.1.

Table 8.1 Minority causes of leg ulcers

Neuropathy: often associated with diabetes mellitus (see Q8.18)

Malignancy: basal cell carcinoma, squamous cell carcinoma or melanoma (see Q8.21 and Q11.1)

Infections: tuberculosis, deep fungal infections, leprosy, syphilis. These are rare in the UK but do consider, particularly if the patient has been travelling or living in the tropics

Lymphoedema: usually only associated with ulceration following cellulitis (see Q10.5) or if venous disease is also present (Morison 1991)

Blood disorders: e.g. sickle-cell disease, thalassaemia

Self-inflicted ulcers

Iatrogenic: these can be caused by ill-fitting plaster casts or badly applied bandages being used to treat existing ulcers

Q8.4   What are the clinical signs and symptoms of chronic venous hypertension?

Signs of venous disease include the following:

- Varicose veins
- Lipodermatosclerosis: hardening of the dermis and subcutaneous fat (see Figure 1.1)
- Stasis eczema
- Ankle flare: the appearance of many dilated intradermal venules over the medial aspect of the ankle
- Staining of the skin as a result of breakdown products of haemo-globin from extravasated red blood cells.
- Atrophe blanche: areas of white skin with tiny spots that are dilated capillary loops (see Q8.14).

Q8.5   What is a typical medical history of a patient with venous disease?

A medical history of patients with venous disease may include any of the following:

- Varicose veins (either treated or untreated) (see Q8.14)
- Deep vein thrombosis

- Phlebitis of the affected leg
- Suspected deep vein thrombosis, e.g. swollen leg after surgery, pregnancy or trauma
- Surgery on affected leg
- Trauma to the affected leg, e.g. fracture
- History of pulmonary embolism.

Q8.6   What is the typical appearance of a venous ulcer?

The following are typical of a venous ulcer:

- Site: often near the medial or lateral malleolus.
- Depth and shape: usually shallow with a poorly defined edge.
- Pain: the pain of venous ulceration is often associated with oedema, from local infections or cellulitis (see Q10.5). Pain is usually relieved by compression bandaging and elevation (see Q8.29).
- Development: usually slow unless infected (see Q10.1).

Q8.7   What are the clinical signs and symptoms of arterial disease?

Signs of arterial disease may include the following:

- Cold legs and feet in a warm environment
- Pale or blue feet when raised
- Feet dusky pink when unsupported
- Shiny hairless leg
- Gangrenous toes
- Absent foot pulses
- Trophic changes to nails
- Poor tissue perfusion; if the nail bed has direct pressure applied to it, it takes longer than 3 seconds to return to normal colour.

Q8.8   What is the typical medical history of a patient with arterial disease?

A medical history suggestive of arterial involvement may include the following:

- Hypertension
- Myocardial infarction

- Angina
- Transient ischaemic attacks
- Arterial surgery
- Cerebrovascular accident (see Q8.15)
- Intermittent claudication (see Q8.15)
- Rheumatoid arthritis (see Q8.16)
- Diabetes mellitus (see Q8.18)
- Peripheral vascular disease (see Q8.18).

Q8.9 What is the typical appearance of an arterial ulcer?

The following are typical of arterial ulcers:

- Site: often on the foot or lateral aspect of the leg but may occur anywhere including the malleolar areas.
- Depth and shape: often deep with a punched-out appearance, often irregular shapes or multiple small areas.
- Pain: invariably painful, often the pain is made worse by elevation or exercise. Patient may report hanging the legs out of bed to relieve pain.
- Development: often rapid.

Q8.10 What should be included in the assessment of a patient presenting with leg ulcers?

Successful treatment of leg ulcers requires thorough assessment to allow the diagnosis of the underlying pathology. Assessment should include assessment of the patient's general condition, ulcer-related history, clinical investigations and examination of the ulcer itself.

Patient assessment and wound assessment have been discussed in some detail in earlier questions, but an overview and issues specific to leg ulcers are given in Table 8.2. (see Q2.1–Q2.4 and Q2.14).

Ulcer-related history

The assessment of a patient presenting with either a first or a recurrent leg ulcer should include a detailed history of the onset of the problems. Q8.4–Q8.6 describe the clinical signs and symptoms, appearance of the ulcer and relevant medical history.

Table 8.2 Assessment of the patient's general condition

Assessment should include:

Age

Sex

Family history: there may be a predisposing factor in leg ulcer development

Occupational history: venous leg ulcers are often associated with occupations involving
    prolonged standing

Mobility: reduced mobility contributes to ulcer development and poor healing (see
    Q8.14)

Diet: poor nutritional status may delay healing (see Q3.4)

Obesity: may contribute to poor healing and ulcer development (see Q3.4)

Smoking habits: may contribute to poor healing and circulatory disease (see Q3.9 and
    Q8.15)

General living conditions

Psychological status: this is important in determining a patient's participation in care
    and his or her compliance with treatment

The patient should have a thorough examination of both the legs, whether or not ulcerated. Any history of ulceration should be included, with duration, treatments used or known allergies to dressings (see Q5.20). A history of the current episode of ulceration should also be documented.

Q8.11 What clinical investigations may be necessary?

Some routine investigations can aid the diagnosis of the leg ulcer or help in its management. Other investigations will be necessary only in a few circumstances. Investigations are summarised in Table 8.3.

Table 8.3 Clinical investigations

Investigation	Rationale
Blood pressure measurement	To detect hypertension (see Q8.8)
Urinalysis/BM stick	To detect diabetes (see Q8.8)
Blood tests	Full blood count and haemoglobin levels to identify anaemia. Test for rheumatoid factor (see Q3.4 and Q8.8)
Wound swab	If signs of infection are present, to determine antibiotic sensitivity (see Q10.1)
Tissue biopsy	If malignancy is suspected (see Table 8.1)
Weight	If the patient is obese, dietary advice and weight reduction can aid healing (see Q3.4)

Q8.12 How can vascular status be assessed?

The simplest form of vascular assessment is to palpate the foot pulses, both the dorsalis pedis and the posterior tibial (Figure 8.1).

However, the presence of oedema may make these pulses difficult to feel. A more accurate way to ascertain the condition of the arterial circulation is to measure the ankle brachial pressure index (ABPI) using Doppler ultrasonography. This should be done only by a nurse who has received training and practised under supervision. The brief description given here is not sufficient to enable anyone to start using this technique.

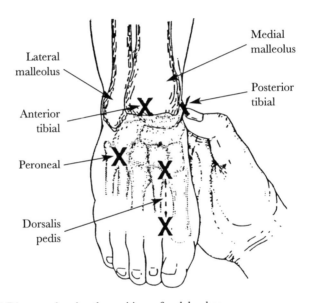

Figure 8.1 Diagram showing the positions of pedal pulses.

Measuring the ankle brachial pressure index

This determines the ratio of the ankle to the brachial systolic pressure with the aid of a battery-operated hand-held Doppler probe.

The patient should be lying as flat as possible for at least 10 minutes (Morison and Moffatt 1994). This is to overcome the effects of exercise on the blood pressure. This time can be used to take the patient's history.

The brachial systolic should be recorded for both arms and the higher figure used for calculation (Vowden et al. 1996). An appropriately sized sphygmomanometer cuff is placed around the arm and ultrasound gel placed over the brachial pulse to ensure a good seal between the probe and the skin. The Doppler probe is placed at a slight angle over the brachial pulse until a good signal is heard. The cuff is inflated until the signal disappears and then gradually deflated until the signal returns. This is the brachial systolic pressure.

To take the foot pulses, secure an appropriately sized sphygmomanometer cuff just above the medial malleolus. Any wounds will require covering to prevent contamination either to or from the cuff. In turn, locate the dorsalis pedis, posterior tibial and anterior tibial pulses. For each pulse inflate the cuff until the signal is lost, then slowly deflate the cuff until the signal returns. For maximum accuracy each pulse should be measured twice. It should be noted that the dorsalis pedis pulse is congenitally absent in up to 12% of people (Barnhorst and Barner 1968).

In practice it is often necessary to use only two of the pedal pulses for measurement (Moffatt 1998). If there is any doubt whatsoever about the patient's arterial status, advice should be sought from a specialist.

To calculate the ABPI divide the highest ankle pressure measured by the highest brachial pressure.

Ankle systolic pressure/Brachial systolic pressure = Ankle brachial pressure index

The value obtained for the ABPI should normally be greater than 1.0. If the reading obtained is below 1.0 some degree of arterial disease is indicated. An ABPI of 0.80–0.95 would indicate minor levels of arterial disease. An ABPI below 0.8 indicates significant arterial disease and compression bandaging is contraindicated. Referral for further vascular assessment is required (Morison and Moffatt 1994). A ratio of 0.50–0.75 will often mean that the patient suffers intermittent claudication, and below this level ischaemic rest pain which will require rapid referral to a vascular surgeon (see Q8.13).

An ABPI of over 1.2 may be pathological, e.g. patients with diabetes may show a falsely high ABPI as a result of medicinal calcinosis, with vessels being difficult to compress. Compression bandages should not be applied to people with diabetes except under close medical supervision (Morison and Moffatt 1994) (see Q8.18).

If there is any doubt about the significance of an ABPI, a doctor should be consulted for advice. No one who has not been trained to do Doppler readings should attempt this procedure. Contact the local tissue viability nurse, wound care nurse or district nurse manager for advice.

Doppler readings should be carried out when the patient first presents with an episode of ulceration, if the ulcer is deteriorating or if the ulcer does not respond to treatment after 3 months and at regular intervals during treatment, e.g. 6 monthly.

Q8.13 When should the patient be referred to another professional?

The vast majority of ulcers should not require specialist assessment. In some instances, further advice and assessment may be required, e.g.:

- A significantly reduced ABPI. Discuss with the GP the need for vascular referral (see Q8.12).
- Rapid deterioration of the ulcer.
- Suspected malignancy (see Q8.21).
- Newly diagnosed diabetes mellitus (see Q3.3 and Q8.18).
- Signs of contact dermatitis (see Q5.20).
- Cellulitus (see Q10.5).
- Ulcers that fail to respond to treatment after a 3-month period (see Q8.32).

Some areas may have specialist nurses who may be able to give advice in these instances; other areas will be dependent on consultant referral.

Q8.14 How does venous disease cause ulceration?

The venous system in the leg comprises both deep and superficial veins (Figure 8.2). The deep veins are the popliteal and femoral veins. The superficial veins are the long and short saphenous veins which lie outside the deep fascia.

Q8.17 How should ulcers associated with rheumatoid arthritis be managed?

This depends on the underlying cause of the ulcer (see Q8.2 and Q8.3), and the treatment should be based on this. If the cause is chronic venous hypertension, graduated compression should be applied but it is extremely important to exclude arterial disease (see Q8.12 and Q8.29).

Particular attention should be given to the skin to prevent further deterioration or trauma. The skin should be kept supple and treated with emollients (see Q4.5), and if adhesive dressings are used great care must be taken in removing them so as not to damage the skin further.

Many of these patients have a poor appetite (Morison and Moffatt 1994) and may require nutritional supplements (see Q3.4–Q3.7).

Regular ankle and foot exercises will be of benefit but the patient may require help with these (see Q8.29).

Oedema may be a problem for patients who cannot raise their legs as a result of arthritic changes or coexisting peripheral vascular disease.

Q8.18 Why are patients with diabetes mellitus prone to ulceration?

Patients with diabetes may develop ulcers as a result of one or a combination of underlying pathologies, so careful assessment of the patient is vital.

Ulceration of the lower limb, particularly the foot, is very common in patients with diabetes mellitus. They have delayed healing and an increased risk of infection (Joseph and Axler 1990). Gangrene may develop leading to lower limb amputation.

Diabetic foot ulcers may result from peripheral neuropathy, peripheral vascular insufficiency and infection, either singly or as a combination.

Peripheral vascular disease is common in people with diabetes, and tends to occur more rapidly and at a younger age (Levin 1988). Calcification of the blood vessels is also significant in people with diabetes.

Risk factors increasing the risk of vascular disease are increasing age, duration of diabetes, smoking, hypertension and hypercholesterolaemia (Morison and Moffatt 1994).

People with diabetes may also have changes to small vessels as well as the larger arteries. This means that the toes may suffer ischaemic damage. This risk is much greater in people with poorly controlled diabetes.

Other diabetic ulcers are the result of neuropathy. There are three types of neuropathy: sensory, motor and autonomic. People with diabetes and sensory neuropathy have reduced or absent pain sensations in their feet, which can lead to unnoticed damage. This can be mechanical, e.g. standing on a sharp object or shoes rubbing, thermal, e.g. scalding from standing in water that is too hot, or chemical, e.g. from self-treatment with chemical corn removers.

Motor neuropathy results in foot deformity with clawing of the toes and metatarsal heads. This changes the patient's gait and produces unnatural pressure, which may result in a build-up of callus and ulceration on the sole of the foot, especially over areas such as the first metatarsal head, enlarged bunions and bony prominences on the toes.

Autonomic neuropathy results in the absence of sweating which means that the skin becomes very dry and prone to develop cracks and fissures that allow the entry of fungi and bacteria. Unlike most ulcers of the skin, these ulcers develop initially from deep within the tissues. Fluid collects under callus formation and becomes infected, leading to abscess formation and ulceration (Morison and Moffatt 1994). The opening of the ulcer may be small and the extent of the tissue damage not immediately obvious. This can lead to further infection extending down to the tendon and bone. If treatment is not rapid, radical débridement may be required (see Q2.10, Q5.11 and Q5.15)

Although people with diabetes are prone to the types of ulcer described here, they may also present with venous ulceration or some of the more rare types of ulcer. As a group, it is especially important that patients with diabetes have the underlying cause of their ulcer determined as soon as possible (see Q8.12); they have a particular need for specialist vascular assessment.

Q8.19 What advice should patients with diabetes be given about foot care?

This advice is probably best given both verbally and with a leaflet that the patient can keep for reference (Box 8.1).

Box 8.1 Foot care advice for people with diabetes

Wash feet daily, making sure they dry them well particularly between the toes

Feet should be checked daily for any damage, redness or blistering. If patients cannot see their own feet, they should ask a carer or friend to do this. Any minor injuries should be reported to the GP immediately

Socks and stockings should be clean and changed daily

Footwear should be checked for foreign bodies such as stones and felt for any jagged edges, before wear

New shoes should be fitted by a trained fitter

Care of toenails, callus and corns should be performed by a podiatrist, who should be informed that the patient has diabetes

Patients should be aware of extreme temperatures and check the temperature of the bath before putting their feet in. They should also try to keep the feet warm to avoid chilblains which may ulcerate

Patients should be asked not to wear socks or stockings with bulky seams or darns that may dig in, and not to wear shoes without socks or stockings

Patients should not walk bare foot

Patients should not perform their own podiatry or use chemicals to remove corns or callus

Patients should not to put their feet too close to the fire, put their feet on hot water bottles or soak their feet for a long time

Patients should avoid tight corsets and garters which will restrict blood flow to the lower limbs

They should not smoke

Q8.20 Should diabetic ulcers be managed like other arterial ulcers?

Although many ulcers on patients with diabetes are the result of arterial problems, their special needs should be borne in mind.

They should have a speedy referral for specialist treatment so that the ulcer does not deteriorate rapidly and lead to lower limb amputation (see Q8.13).

The care is most effective when it is multidisciplinary, involving the physician, specialist diabetic nurse, podiatrist, orthotist and, in some cases, the vascular and orthopaedic surgeon (Morison and Moffatt 1994).

Levin (1988) suggests that the management of diabetic foot ulcers should be aggressive. This involves rapid local débridement leaving only healthy tissue, systemic antibiotic therapy, diabetic control and non-weight-bearing for plantar ulcers.

An appropriate local dressing should be chosen but the ulcer will respond only if the above treatment is given. However, an inappropriate dressing may make the situation worse.

Ulcerated feet/toes should be kept dry to eliminate maceration between the toes which will allow infections to enter (see Q5.1). Patients should be given advice about foot care (see Box 8.1).

The person with diabetes should be strongly advised to stop smoking and to follow dietary advice to reduce long-term complications.

For further information about management of diabetes, the reader is referred to Turner and Crosby, *Diabetes: A Handbook for Community Nurses* – in this series.

Q8. 21 When should I suspect that an ulcer is malignant?

Malignant ulcers are rare in the UK (more frequent in tropical countries), but if ulcers fail to respond to treatment this should not be overlooked as a cause (Ackroyd and Young 1983).

Squamous cell carcinoma may develop in a chronic venous ulcer (it then becomes known as a Marjolin's ulcer). Although uncommon, it may be suspected if the ulcer has an unusual appearance with overgrowth of tissue at the base of the wound or wound margins. Confirmation is by biopsy and histological examination.

Melanomas are more common but unlikely to be mistaken for venous ulceration.

Kaposi's sarcomas are again rare, but becoming more common with the spread of acquired immune deficiency syndrome (AIDS); they are usually small and multiple and may ulcerate (Morison and Moffatt 1994).

Q8.22 What are the main aims of leg ulcer treatment?

The aim of treatment is threefold:

1. To heal the ulcer
2. To treat the underlying condition
3. To prevent reoccurrence.

Q8.23 What primary dressings should be used on leg ulcers?

Choice of dressing will depend on the wound state (see Chapter 5). In most instances a simple dressing that is capable of maintaining a moist, warm environment conducive to wound healing should be chosen (see Q5.8). Excessive exudate should be absorbed. Dressings should be non-toxic, non-adherent, non-allergenic and non-sensitising (Morgan 1987). Under four-layer compression bandages, often all that is necessary is a simple non-adherent dressing (see Q8.29).

Q8.24 How often should the dressing be changed?

Unless there is excessive exudate, discomfort or bandage slippage, the dressing should be changed once a week (NHS Executive 1995). However, the treatment regimen should be determined in conjunction with the patient and there will be instances where more frequent changes are necessary.

Q8.25 What is the best way to cleanse an ulcer?

Ulcers should be cleansed by irrigation with warm physiological saline if necessary (see Q4.3 and Q4.4). If there is no old dressing material or exudate this may not be needed. Legs may be washed with warm tap water containing an emollient if desired. If using a communal bucket, it should be lined with plastic (new for each patient) and cleansed between use by local infection control methods, to prevent any cross-infection. Washing helps to keep the skin in good condition by removing loose skin scales and is also pleasant for the patient who may otherwise be unable to wash the feet and legs for long periods.

Q8.26 Some patients with leg ulcers seem sensitive to the products used. How can this be avoided or treated?

Patients can become sensitised to treatments at any time (see Q5.20 and Q5.21). Patients with reactions to unknown sensitisers should be referred to a dermatologist for patch testing. In cases of sensitivity, remove the known or potential allergen, apply a simple non-adherent dressing, and elevate and rest the limb. Liaise with the GP to prescribe a steroid ointment (cream may contain sensitisers). Apply the ointment for 2–4 days. Reduce the amount of ointment used over the following 3–4 days and replace the steroid with white soft paraffin emollient.

Q8.27 Some leg ulcers are very painful. Is there anything practical that can be done to help?

If the pain is at the wound site, consider whether the dressing is causing the discomfort. It may be sticking to the wound and causing trauma when the patient moves. A less adherent dressing would reduce the pain. Or, if the dressing is very hydrophilic and causing a stinging or drawing sensation on the wound bed, again changing to a product more suitable to the wound will help (see Q2.7).

Compression therapy, exercise and elevation will reduce oedema and pain in patients with venous ulceration (see Q8.29).

Analgesia must be tailored to the individual patient's requirements; in cases such as arterial ulceration when pain may be severe, opiate analgesia may be required (see Q2.7–Q2.9).

Q8.28 What should patients be offered in terms of education?

All patients should be offered accessible and appropriate information on their leg ulcer disease. This should include the rationale for their treatment, self-help strategies, services available to them, dietary advice and lifestyle advice. Patients with any type of ulcer should be encouraged to exercise because mobilising will encourage venous return and limit the effects of immobility (Morison and Moffatt 1994), but their capabilities will vary (see Q8.29). Many manufacturing companies produce comprehensive patient booklets which can be obtained from representatives. Consider using your own educational and health promotional skills.

Q8.29 How should venous ulcers be treated?

The underlying venous disease must be treated. This is the most important aspect of treatment and unless this is made a priority the ulcer is unlikely to respond to local treatment.

If arterial involvement has been excluded (see Q8.12), the underlying venous disorder should be treated with compression bandaging, exercise and elevation.

Compression

Graduated compression will assist venous return and improve muscle pump function. The suggested level of compression is between 20 and 40 mmHg at the ankle, to 50% of that value at the knee (Kendrick et al. 1994). A compression bandage should be anchored at the base of the toes, exert maximum compression at the ankle and finish at the knee.

Manufacturers' instructions should be followed. Bandages that are incorrectly applied are at best uncomfortable and useless and at worst dangerous. It is important that anyone applying a compression bandage has been taught the correct method of application, understands the rationale for the treatment and is competent to carry out the treatment.

Compression can be applied as a single-layer, long, stretch bandage, e.g. SurePress or Tensopress. Orthopaedic padding may be required to protect the leg, particularly over bony prominences. Note that patients with an ankle circumference of less than 18 cm (see Figure 8.3, p. 76) are not suitable for compression unless sufficient padding is applied to build up the ankle size.

Multilayer compression systems (again using long stretch bandages) provide adequate padding and adequate sustained compression for at least a week. In most instances, a weekly dressing change is recommended. Only accepted systems should be used. These may come in kit form, e.g. Profore or Ultra Four or bandages can be purchased separately. All patients should have their ankle circumference measured to ensure that the appropriate bandage regimen is selected. Manufacturers' instructions for application should be adhered to and the practitioner appropriately trained in the application of multilayer bandaging.

Alternatively, short stretch bandages can be used, e.g. Comprilan, Rosidal K. These have been used effectively in Europe since the early 1960s. They are 100% cotton (useful if the patient is allergic to elastic fibres – see Q5.20). They are applied at full stretch so that during exercise to the calf muscle the bandage does not expand in the way a long stretch bandage would. The working force of the calf muscle is therefore reflected back into the leg (Charles 1999). When washed they have no elasticity to lose and can be reused with the same effect as when new. Padding should be used over areas prone to pressure damage such as the Achilles' tendon, bunion area, tibia, malleoli and the dorsum of the foot. Initially, when used oedema reduces so the bandage will need reapplying as the leg circumference reduces, otherwise any benefits will be lost.

Exercise

Walking exercises the calf muscle and works the muscle pump, increasing venous return. Many patients with venous ulcers are capable of a mile or more; this should be encouraged. However, if they are elderly or have other disabilities, this will not be achievable; advice should be tailored to suit the patient's capabilities. Regular flexion and extension exercises are beneficial in working the calf muscle pump for patients with limited mobility.

Elevation

Patients should be encouraged to elevate their legs above hip height when sitting to facilitate venous return.

Q8.30 How should mixed aetiology or arterial ulcers be treated?

If the ABPI is between 0.8 and 0.95, the limb can have compression therapy (see Q8.12). Below this level, unless advised to the contrary, e.g. by a vascular surgeon, ulcers should be treated as arterial.

Q8.31 What is the recommended management for arterial ulceration?

Compression must not be used on ulcers with a substantial arterial component. Any bandages used should be light retention bandages. Mild exercise and ankle exercises should be encouraged especially if the patient is immobile (see Q8.29). Severe arterial disease may restrict mobility to less than 100 yards.

Pain control may be achieved by rest, analgesia and a suitable dressing, e.g. foam, hydrogel or hydrocolloid (see Q2.7–Q2.9 and Q5.13–Q5.16).

Patients with arterial disease, particularly those with an ABPI below 0.75, should be considered for a surgical opinion (see Q8.12).

Q8.32 When does a trauma to the leg become an ulcer?

If the patient has a history of leg ulceration and known vascular problems, any minor injury to the leg should be treated as a recurrence of ulceration, and appropriate treatment commenced immediately (see Q2.3 and Q8.10).

In other patients, if the wound does not respond as you would expect other minor wounds to, a vascular assessment should be carried out and if either venous or arterial disease is discovered the wound should be treated as an ulcer (see Q8.12).

People without vascular problems may still have problems with more major knocks; even in healthy people the skin over the tibia is poorly vascularised and pretibial lacerations can take some time to heal (see Q7.8).

Q8.33 When should the treatment be changed?

Individual healing rates will vary whatever the underlying condition. Any ulcer not responding to treatment in 4–8 weeks should be reassessed. Treatment may need to be changed or the patient may require further investigation or referral to a specialist nurse or consultant (see Q8.13).

Q8.34 How can recurrence be prevented?

Approximately 75% of patients suffer recurrence of ulceration. This can be reduced if appropriate advice is given.

Patients should be advised to report any new damage to legs as soon as possible, so that treatment can be started. Patients with venous disease require compression for life. When healing is complete, they should be measured for suitable hosiery (see Q8.35–Q8.41).

Encourage patients to continue with exercise (see Q8.29). Reinforce advice on diet, lifestyle and smoking habits. Encourage protection of the legs from trauma damage and continue to monitor the underlying disease.

Q8.35 What is the role of compression hosiery in preventing recurrence of venous ulceration?

As the primary cause of venous ulceration is the development of pathological venous hypertension, it is important that the underlying cause continues to be treated (see Q8.14 and Q8.29).

Graduated compression hosiery applies external pressure to the skin and underlying tissues which supports the superficial veins, helping to counteract the raised capillary pressure and thus reducing oedema. The reduction of oedema has been shown to be a crucial factor in relation to both ulcer healing and preventing further skin breakdown and ulceration (Moffatt and O'Hare 1995).

Q8.36 Which are preferred – above- or below-knee stockings?

For most patients either length is equally effective (Moffatt and O'Hare 1995). However, above-knee stockings are more appropriate if oedema collects around the knee, or if the patient has arthritic changes to the knee that cause below-knee stockings to be uncomfortable.

In other patients, compliance may be more likely with below-knee stockings which are relatively easy to put on. Although class 3 stockings (compression 25–35 mmHg) are desirable, a patient with dexterity problems may be encouraged to comply by moving down to class 2 (compression 18–24 mmHg).

Q8.37 Should stockings be open or closed toe?

This is a question of patient preference. Some patients, especially those with deformities of the toe such as hammer toes, find closed stockings uncomfortable and restrictive, whereas others find open toes dig in where the stocking ends.

Q8.38 What measurements should be taken before ordering stockings?

Measuring the limb accurately is important so that the stocking is fitted properly and to ensure comfort. Ill-fitting, uncomfortable stockings reduce patient compliance in regular wearing of the stocking.

Measurements should be taken either first thing in the morning before any oedema has accumulated or immediately after the ulcer has healed and the compression bandage has been removed.

Most patients will fit into the standard sizes available on prescription but those with very long or disproportionate legs may require made-to-measure stockings. If both legs require a stocking they should be measured separately. The measurements required are shown in Figure 8.3.

Manufacturers suggest that stockings should be renewed every 6 months. The limb should be measured on each occasion that a

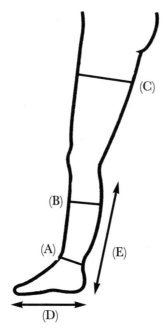

Figure 8.3 Measurements to be taken when fitting compression stockings. (A) The ankle at its narrowest point; (B) the calf at its widest point; (C) above knee only: the thigh at its widest point; (D) the length of the foot; (E) length of leg, heel to below knee. The patient should be bare legged and standing to ensure accurate measurement.

stocking is required. It may be preferable to keep the patient in compression bandages for 3–4 weeks after healing to limit the possibility of damage to newly formed fragile skin.

Q8.39 There are different classes of compression hosiery. What are their uses?

Compression hosiery falls into three classes.

- Class 1: gives 14–17 mmHg pressure at the ankle. They are recommended for varicose veins and mild oedema.
- Class 2: gives 18–23 mmHg pressure at the ankle. They are recommended for moderate-to-severe varicose veins and prevention of ulcer reoccurrence.
- Class 3: gives 25–35 mmHg pressure at the ankle. They are recommended for gross varices, postphlebitic legs, recurrent ulceration and lymphoedema.

A class 3 stocking is the best choice for patients with repeated episodes of ulceration and considerable venous disease but they are difficult to put on, particularly for elderly patients. Generally a class 2 stocking is recognised as sufficient to prevent recurrence if venous disease is not severe, although there is little available research in this area (Moffatt and O'Hare 1995).

If a patient has very limited dexterity two class 1 stockings may prove easier to put on (this will give greater pressure than a class 2 overall).

Q8.40 Are there any tips for easier application of hosiery?

Some aids are available to assist with application such as the Valet (Medi) but these are not available on prescription and have to be purchased from a pharmacy.

Patients may find application easier if they dust their leg lightly with a simple non-perfumed talcum powder before application to make the stocking slip on more easily. Wearing rubber gloves may help to grip the stocking. For open-toed stockings, placing a Chinese slipper or plastic bag over the foot may aid pulling the stocking over the foot. The bag or slipper should be pulled out once the stocking is in place.

Q8.41 Are there any hazards associated with the use of compression stockings?

The biggest hazard is if the patient has a significant amount of arterial disease (see Q8.12). Careful patient assessment, preferably with a Doppler probe, should eliminate this problem. For the patient with arterial disease, the development of pressure necrosis is a potential hazard.

Ill-fitting stockings may also cause pressure or friction damage, particularly over the tibial crest, the dorsum of the foot, the bunion area, overcrowded or deformed toes or any ankle deformity.

Stockings should be checked for correct fit around arthritic deformed knees where they may form constricting cuffs, giving a tourniquet effect. Some patients may suffer from skin allergies or irritation (see Q5.20) and will require a stocking that has a cotton layer next to the leg.

Q8.42 How can patients be prevented from interfering with their ulcers, thus delaying healing?

Much has been written about the 'social ulcer' but the actual number of patients who interfere with their ulcer in an attempt to delay healing is unknown. Some patients may interfere with their bandages for a good reason, e.g.:

- The compression bandage may have been applied unevenly up the leg, causing ridges in the skin that are painful.
- The bandage may have been applied too tightly, causing pain.
- If the bandage has slipped, it may feel uncomfortable or form a tight band, causing swelling over the top.
- The patient may have problems getting shoes and socks on without disturbing the bandage.
- If the leg is itchy, the patient may be using something like a knitting needle to scratch the itch.

All of these issues should be considered before suspecting the patient of interfering to intentionally delay healing. If this is in fact the problem, it needs to be dealt with gently. Many of these patients are elderly and lonely, and enjoy social contact with the nurse. One way of ensuring contact is to hold 'well ulcer' clinics (see Q8.43).

Q8.43 What is a 'well ulcer' clinic?

These clinics have been shown to reduce recurrence rates (Morison and Moffat 1994). They can be used to reiterate advice (see Q8.28). Support stockings can be checked and renewed if necessary (see Q8.38). The legs can be checked for skin condition and any knocks the patient may not have noticed. Appropriate treatment can be commenced immediately.

The following three scenarios illustrate a few of the aspects of leg ulcer care.

Case study 4

Mrs B was an active woman in her mid-40s who worked as a school dinner lady, and enjoyed activities such as line dancing.

Twelve months previously she had developed a small leg ulcer and attended the GP's surgery. He prescribed tulle dressings and

Tubigrip and asked her to do her own dressings. During this year, the leg had failed to respond to the treatment and the ulcer had slightly increased in size. She was also feeling miserable, because the pain from her ulcer was stopping her enjoying line dancing, and she felt unattractive.

Finally she decided to seek a second opinion. At assessment, her ulcer was shown to be venous. It measured approximately 3 × 4 cm and was covered by approximately 50% slough. Four-layer compression was commenced and she agreed to take 1 month off work to stop the necessity for prolonged standing. After 1 week she was reviewed. The ulcer had started to reduce in size and was now 2 × 3.5 cm with about 25% slough. She also felt more comfortable. Within another 3 weeks the ulcer measured 1 × 1.5 cm and was clean. Fortunately, 2 weeks later (school holidays) saw the ulcer healed.

She was amazed at the progress and happy to wear the prescribed stockings. She was less happy about the wasted year of treatment.

Case study 5

Mrs L had had a venous ulcer for 2 years. Despite compression therapy and appropriate dressings, it remained static and the nursing team, while frustrated at the lack of progress, were resigned to twice-weekly dressing changes.

One team member started a developmental course and began to question what was best practice. She decided to look at a few patients who failed to respond to treatment and see whether, by reading more about their conditions, she could solve any of the problems. As part of this, she started to read about wound healing and realised that, although the compression therapy and dressings were fine, there could be some other underlying pathology preventing ulcer healing. She persuaded the team leader to take a blood sample from Mrs L, and the results showed pernicious anaemia. Appropriate treatment was commenced by the GP and after a few months the ulcer slowly started to improve.

Case study 6

Mr F was an active 86-year-old man. He lived alone with no help and each day cycled to the shops or working men's club. He enjoyed other people's company and was happy. He had a 12-year history of bilateral venous ulceration about which he seemed to be unperturbed.

They appeared to cause him no discomfort and although extensive they were static, not changing in size from month to month. The ulcers were dressed three times a week by the district nurse.

As the nurses gained a better understanding of the benefits of compression therapy, they decided to start Mr F on compression bandaging. An improvement in condition could be seen very quickly. However, Mr F became progressively more irritable and miserable. It transpired that he felt the bandages were impeding his cycling. He was relying on neighbours doing his shopping and errands, and he had been unable to go on his regular visits to the club. Mr F was persuaded to get his bicycle out and demonstrate the problem. It was apparent that, whether or not it was a practical or psychological problem, he was unable to cycle. He persevered for a further 2 weeks getting visibly lower in mood. The nurse met with the health-care team to discuss the problem. The team were divided. Half felt that the new regimen was reducing the frequency of visits and thus costs and, as there was an improvement, compression should continue. Half felt that his rapid decline in his general condition and mood offset any benefits and that isolating him was inappropriate.

What would you do?

P.S. Called in to adjudicate I decided that given his age and that the size of the ulcers would preclude fast healing, to make an old man happy, we should let him live with his ulcers and ride his bike.

Summary

There are several causes of leg ulceration and it is important to determine ulcer type at the onset of treatment. Thorough assessment of the patient's general condition, the affected limb, ulcer site and a vascular assessment are essential. The aim of treatment is threefold: to heal the ulcer, to treat the underlying condition and to prevent reoccurrence.

CHAPTER 9

Pressure sores

Pressure ulcers are a common problem. Incidence and prevalence studies generally demonstrate that between 3% and 10% of the population in both hospital and community settings acquire a degree of pressure damage while undergoing care (Land 1994), although some estimates put the figure higher. Financial costs to the NHS have been estimated as high as £775 million a year (West and Priestley 1994). This includes staff time, drugs, dressings and hospital overheads, but excludes costs to the patient such as pain, suffering, loss of independence and in some circumstances life. These costs are impossible to calculate. It has been estimated that 60 000 deaths a year result from complications of pressure damage, although death certificates rarely reflect this (Staas and Cioschi 1991).

Patients are becoming increasingly concerned about pressure sores being an unnecessary complication of medical treatment and are beginning to seek recompense through the courts. In 1987 damages of £100 000 were awarded to a successful claimant (Silver 1987).

It is obvious that the prevention of pressure ulcers should be of paramount importance to the nurse. However, it is apparent that not all pressure sore development is preventable. Loader et al. (1994) estimate that, although 95% of pressure damage can be avoided, the remaining 5% is inevitable, resulting from factors such as damage being present before the care episode, debilitating underlying conditions and extraordinary circumstances.

Although nurses do not work in isolation, nursing care must be regarded as a major influence on outcomes related to pressure area care.

Q9.1   How is a pressure sore defined?

The European Pressure Ulcer Advisory Panel 1997 (EPUAP) gives a working definition as:

> A pressure ulcer is an area of localised damage to the skin and underlying tissue caused by pressure, shear, friction and/or a combination of these.

Q9.2   What is meant by the prevalence and incidence of pressure ulcers?

It is important to know the rates of prevalence and incidence as a baseline so that improvements can be monitored.

Prevalence

Dealey (1993) defines prevalence as 'the measurement of the number of persons with a specific disease or condition from within a given population, measured at a particular point in time'. Thus these studies give a 'snapshot' of the situation and can be used to demonstrate the effectiveness of prevention strategies and used to identify any additional resources that are required. Prevalence studies do not differentiate between where sores are acquired.

Incidence

Incidence is: 'the number of persons developing a specific disease or condition as a proportion of the local population, measured over a period of time' (Dealey 1993).
   Incidence studies are more detailed and include outcomes. They are more time-consuming to complete than prevalence studies and require regular data collection, and rely heavily on staff motivation.

Q9.3   What are the causes of pressure ulcers?

The causes of pressure ulcers can be divided into:

•   intrinsic factors (conditions inherent in the patient)
•   extrinsic factors (conditions outside the patient).

Q9.4   What are the intrinsic factors that cause pressure ulcers?

Intrinsic factors that cause pressure ulcers include the following:

Gender

The Waterlow (1985) risk assessment tool takes gender into account and shows women to be at greater risk of pressure damage than men. However, the reasons are poorly understood.

Age

Pressure damage can occur at any age but is more common in elderly people because skin has lost elasticity and they are more likely to have concurrent diseases (Nyquist and Hawthorne 1987).

Immobility

A reduction in mobility for any reason increases the risk of developing pressure damage (Dealey 1994).

Body weight

Low body weight gives less protection from pressure over bony prominences. Obese patients may sweat, increasing the risk of shear or friction (Dealey 1994).

Nutrition

Malnutrition is a primary contributing factor and reduces the tissue's ability to withstand pressure (Makleburst and Siegreen 1996). It also causes delayed healing (McLaren 1992; Dealey 1994) (see also Q3.4–Q3.7). Obese patients can also be malnourished (see Q9.7).

Medication

Steroids, anti-inflammatory drugs, strong analgesics, sedatives, β-blockers and cytotoxic drugs can increase the risk of pressure damage by reducing mobility, sensation, skin integrity and appetite (Banks 1997).

Incontinence

Incontinence of either faeces or urine can result in skin maceration or excoriation. This leads to increased risk of friction damage and increases the risk of infection (Torrance 1983; Dealey 1994) (see

Q9.7). Some drugs such as aperients, diuretics and antibiotics may exacerbate incontinence (Dealey 1994).

Underlying disease

Many underlying diseases contribute to the development of pressure damage. Neurological problems can cause loss of mobility and sensation. Low blood pressure results in a lower external pressure being required to occlude the capillary vessels. Circulatory problems can reduce blood supply to the tissues and impair the removal of waste products. Other conditions increasing the risk of pressure damage include Alzheimer's disease, carcinoma, diabetes, arthritis, gastrointestinal, liver and renal problems (Dealey 1994; Banks 1997).

Skin condition

Tissue paper skin can be the result of ageing or the use of long-term high-dose steroids (see Q3.8). Oedematous skin can also result in a reduced oxygen supply and impaired removal of waste products (Torrance 1983; Dealey 1994).

Infection

Systemic infection can lead to pyrexia, excessive sweating and tissue breakdown (Banks 1997) (see Q10.1 and Q10.2)

Smoking

See Q3.9. Smoking can also result in loss of appetite.

Other factors

These include pain, state of consciousness, psychological factors, sociological factors and who is providing home care (Dealey 1994).

Q9.5	What are the extrinsic factors that cause pressure ulcers?

Extrinsic factors resulting in patients experiencing pressure damage include pressure, shear and friction.

Pressure

Pressure damage usually occurs over the body's bony prominences. When pressure is applied to the skin from the support surface (i.e.

mattress, trolley) it is transmitted through to the bones, and all the tissues in between are compressed and the capillary vessels occluded (Collier 1999a).

There is no agreement as to the length of time local pressure can be exerted before tissue damage begins, or what pressure is required to occlude the capillary vessels. The amount of pressure required may vary between body parts, depending on the local bone, muscle and skin structure (Collier 1999b). Capillaries in the skin run vertical to the surface and are coiled at their bases, limiting the risk of occlusion, but in subcutaneous tissue the vessels lie in the parallel planes of the deep fascia, following the paths of nerves and ligaments (see Figure 1.1). This causes them to be vulnerable to distortion and occlusion from both external pressure and pressure from underlying bony prominences.

Capillary occlusion results in ischaemic changes and tissue necrosis at and around the point of occlusion within the subcutaneous tissues. The vessels in the subcutaneous tissues also give rise to the perforators, which supply the skin, and so deep vessel obstruction is likely to result in ischaemia of both cutaneous and subcutaneous tissue if pressure is sustained (Collier 1999b).

As the damage from pressure is transmitted through to the deeper tissues, external pressure ulcers may indicate that underlying tissue necrosis is already established. This can be seen when an apparently superficial wound is débrided to reveal an underlying cavity or sinus.

Shearing forces

These can be defined as 'a mechanical stress that is parallel to a plane of interest' (Bennett and Lee 1986). If a high level of shear is present, damage can be caused by only half the amount of pressure normally needed to damage tissue.

Shear ulcers occur when the patient's skin adheres to the bed clothes, particularly when in the sitting position and the patient begins to slide down the bed. The deep fascia moves downwards with the skeletal structures as a result of gravitational forces, whereas the sacral fascia remains attached to the sacral dermis. This stretches the dermal microcirculation and unless resolved avulsion of the local capillaries and arterioles occurs, which in turn increases the possibility of local tissue necrosis (Collier 1999b).

Friction

This is the force related to two surfaces moving across one another. If a patient is not moved using recommended moving and handling techniques, but is dragged or pulled across surfaces, friction can disrupt the epidermis and cause an initial break in the skin. This can occur in a community setting if the patient's carers are also elderly or infirm, and they have difficulty lifting the patient, or if care staff are inadequately trained.

Friction damage can also occur as a result of an ill-fitting plaster cast or limb prosthesis.

Q9.6   How can patients at risk of developing pressure damage be identified?

When initiating a preventive strategy it is necessary to identify those patients at risk of developing pressure sores. This can be achieved by using risk assessment tools, which:

• Act as an *aide-mémoire* to carers (Flanagan 1993)
• Help provide quantifiable data for auditing purposes (Flanagan 1993)
• Provide evidence that preventive/treatment plans are based on objective criteria and a specific rationale (Flanagan 1993)
• Aid the rational allocation of limited resources (such as special mattresses) to those most likely to benefit from them (*Effective Health Care Bulletin* 1995)
• Act as case mix adjusters to help make sensible comparisons of pressure sores between units over time (*Effective Health Care Bulletin* 1995).

The first risk assessment scale was the Norton Pressure Sore Risk Assessment Scale (Norton et al. 1962) Many modifications have appeared since. Norton is probably one of the best known and most widely used (Barrett 1987; Davies 1994) but is felt by some to be too simplistic. It is important to choose a scale that is suitable for your area of work. Although all scales have a research-based rationale, they were designed for different purposes and settings. Norton's scale was designed specifically for use with the older person. Some differences are shown in Tables 9.1 and 9.2.

Table 9.1 The Norton Score*

Physical state		Mental state		Activity	
Good	4	Alert	4	Ambulant	4
Fair	3	Apathetic	3	Walks with help	3
Poor	2	Confused	2	Chairbound	2
Very bad	1	Stuporous	1	Bedbound	1

Mobility		Incontinence	
Full	4	None	4
Slightly limited	3	Occasional	3
Very limited	2	Usually urine	2
Immobile	1	Double	1

*The Norton Score can be used to assess the degree of risk of developing pressure sores. It was developed for use with elderly patients. A score of ≤14 indicates vulnerability to pressure sores. A score of ≤12 is high risk.

Table 9.2 Comparison of risk assessment

Risk factor	Norton	Gosnall	Knoll	Waterlow	Braden
Mobility	/	/	/	/	/
Activity	/	/	/	×	/
Nutritional status	×	/	/	/	/
Mental status	/	/	/	×	/
Incontinence/moisture	/	/	/	/	/
General physical condition	/	×	/	/	×
Skin appearance	×	/	×	/	×
Medication	×	/	×	/	×
Friction/shear	×	×	×	×	/
Weight	×	×	×	/	×
Age	×	×	×	/	×
Specific predisposing disease	×	×	/	/	×
Prolonged pressure	×	×	×	/	×

A comparison of pressure sore risk factors used in various risk assessment scales (Flanagan 1993).

The Waterlow score, Table 9.3, is another popular assessment tool, developed in the UK in 1984. It is more complex than the Norton score (Birchall 1993), covers a larger number of risk factors and groups patients into three categories of risk status. It also covers suggestions for care guidelines.

Table 9.3 The Waterlow Pressure Sore Prevention/Treatment Policy. Reproduced with kind permission of Mrs Judy Waterlow

Waterlow Pressure Sore Prevention/Treatment Policy

RING SCORES IN TABLE, ADD TOTAL. SEVERAL SCORES PER CATEGORY CAN BE USED

Build/Weight for Height	*	Skin Type	*	Sex/Age	*	Special Risks	*
Average	0	Healthy	0	Male	1	**Tissue Malnutrition**	*
Above Average	1	Tissue Paper	1	Female	2	e.g. Terminal Cachexia	8
Obese	2	Dry	1	14–49	1	Cardiac Failure	5
Below Average	3	Oedematous	1	50–64	2	Peripheral Vascular Disease	5
		Clammy (Temp↑)	1	65–74	3	Anaemia	2
		Discoloured	2	75–80	4	Smoking	1
		Broken/Spot	3	81+	5		

Continence	*	Mobility	*	Appetite	*	Neurological Deficit	*
Complete/Catheterised	0	Fully	0	Average	0	e.g. Diabetes, M.S., CVA, Motor/Sensory Paraplegia	4–6
Occasionally Incontinent	1	Restless/Fidgety	1	Poor	1		
Cath/Incontinent of Faeces	2	Apathetic	2	N.G. Tube/Fluids only	2	**Major Surgery/Trauma**	*
Doubly Incontinent	3	Restricted	3	NBM/Anorexic	3	Orthopaedic Below Waist, Spinal	5
		Inert/Traction	4			on Table 2 hours	5
		Chairbound	5				
						Medication	*
						Cytotoxics High Dose steroids Anti-Inflammatory	4

Score	10+ A Risk	15+ High Risk	20+ Very High Risk

Remember tissue damage often starts prior to admission, in casualty. A seated patient is also at risk.

Assessment: If the patient falls into any of the risk categories then preventative nursing is required. A combination of good nursing techniques and preventative aids will definitely be necessary.

WOUND CLASSIFICATION
Stirling Pressure Score severity scale (SPSSS)

Stage 0 — No clinical evidence of pressure sore
0.1 — Healed with scarring
0.2 — Tissue damage not assessed as a pressure sore (a) below

Stage 1 — Discoloration of intact skin
1.1 — Non-blanchable erythema with increased local heat
1.2 — Blue/purple/black discoloration — the sore is at least **Stage 1** (a or b)

Stage 2 — Partial thickness skin loss or damage
2.1 — Blister
2.2 — Abrasion
2.3 — Shallow ulcer, no undermining of adjacent tissue
2.4 — Any of these with underlying blue/purple/black discoloration or induration. The sore is at least **Stage 2** (a, b or c+d for **2.3**, +e for **2.4**)

Stage 3 — Full-thickness skin loss involving damage/necrosis of subcutaneous tissue, not extending to underlying bone tendon or joint capsule
3.1 — Crater, without undermining adjacent tissue
3.2 — Crater, with undermining of adjacent tissue
3.3 — Sinus, the full extent of which is uncertain
3.4 — Necrotic tissue masking full extent of damage.
The sore is at least **Stage 3** (b, +/-e, f, g, +h for **3.4**)

Stage 4 — Full-thickness loss with extensive destruction and tissue necrosis extending to underlying bone tendon or capsule
4.1 — Visible exposure of bone tendon or capsule
4.2 — Sinus assessed as extending to same (b+/-e, f, g, h, i)

Guide to types of Dressings/Treatment
a. Semipermeable membrane
b. Hydrocolloid
c. Foam dressing
d. Alginate
e. Hydrogel
f. Alginate rope/ribbon
g. Foam cavity filler
h. Enzymatic debridement
i. Surgical debridement

PREVENTION:
PREVENTATIVE AIDS:

Special Mattress/Bed: 10+ overlays or specialist foam mattresses.
15+ alternating pressure overlays, mattresses and bed systems.
20+ Bed System: Fluidised, bead, low air loss and alternating pressure mattresses.
Note: Preventative aids cover a wide spectrum of specialist features. Efficacy should be judged, if possible, on the basis of independent evidence.

Cushions: No patient should sit in a wheelchair without some form of cushioning. If nothing else is available — use the patient's own pillow.
10+4" Foam cushion.
15+ Specialist cell and/or foam cushion
20+ Cushion capable of adjustment to suit individual patient.

Bed Clothing: Avoid plastic draw sheets, inco pads and tightly tucked in sheets/sheet covers, especially when using Specialist bed and mattress overlay systems.
Use Duvet-plus vapour permeable cover.

NURSING CARE
General: Frequent changes of position, lying/sitting
Use of pillows
Pain Appropriate pain control
Nutrition High protein, vitamins, minerals
Patient Handling: Correct lifting technique – Hoists – Monkey Pole – Transfer Devices
Patient Comfort Aids: Real sheepskins — Bed Cradle
Operating Table
Theatre/A&E Trolley 4" cover plus adequate protection.
Skin Care: General Hygiene, NO rubbing, cover with an appropriate dressing

If treatment is required, first remove pressure

Risk assessment tools should be used as an addition to clinical judgement. The *Effective Health Care Bulletin* (1995) suggests that there is little evidence that using a pressure sore risk scale is better than clinical judgement or that it improves outcomes. However, any tool that can help to assist in identifying at-risk vulnerable patients is valuable when planning care, but any tool is of benefit only if it is used correctly and the patient's at-risk status is reassessed regularly and whenever there is a change in his or her condition.

Q9.7   How can pressure sores be prevented?

Choice of an appropriate support surface is important (see Q9.8) to remove the extrinsic factors significant in the development and delayed healing of pressure ulcers (Morison 1989), as is alleviating the effects of the intrinsic factors contributing to tissue breakdown. (see Q9.4 and Q9.5)

Assess the patient's risk of developing pressure damage when they first come into your care, and reassess regularly or whenever there is a change in the patient's condition, using a reliable and valid assessment tool (see Q9.6).

Incontinence is often associated with pressure sores (Fletcher 1992). Moisture is known to be a factor in increasing pressure damage risk, and wound exudate and perspiration as well as urine may lead to skin maceration (Priest and Clarke 1993). It has also been suggested that faecal incontinence is a more important factor in pressure damage than urinary incontinence (Priest and Clarke 1993). The patient should be cleansed as soon as possible after being incontinent, excessive soap should not be used, avoid the rubbing of delicate skin, and if possible correct the cause of the incontinence (Ek and Boman 1982). Dealey (1995) suggests that the use of a mild cleanser in a spray format, such as the Triple Care System (Smith & Nephew), may reduce pressure sore incidence.

Malnutrition has also been described as one of the most commonly cited factors in the development of pressure damage (Closs 1993) (see Q9.4). If the patient is failing to eat a balanced diet and/or is losing weight, check on the reason why, and arrange practical help such as meals on wheels if necessary and food supplements such as Fresubin (Fresenius) or Ensure (Abbott) for consumption between meals (see Q3.4–Q3.7). Fluid intake should also be monitored.

Inspect high-risk areas regularly for any signs of damage and develop a plan of mobility/turning appropriate to the patient's risk, which keeps him or her off any damaged skin or high-risk sites as much as possible, bearing in mind the patient's need for comfort, sleep, meals and lifestyle. If much of the care is being carried out by relatives or other carers, it is important to involve them in moving the patient, looking for damage and reporting damage straight away. It may help to have carers' information leaflets available to reinforce advice given (see Q8.28).

Q9.8 What should be taken into account when selecting an appropriate support surface?

When selecting a suitable support surface, whether for an individual patient or for a group of patients (such as in a nursing home), the following factors need to be considered:

- Clinical
- Practical
- Financial (Clark and Fletcher 1999).

Clinical considerations

The intrinsic and extrinsic risk factors (see Q9.4 and Q9.5) need to be considered, and also issues such as: What is the patient's risk level?' and 'Is this expected to change? Has damage already occurred? Does the patient have other requirements from a mattress, such as needing a firm edge to allow transfer out of bed? Are there any medical problems that make certain types of mattress unsuitable? (Clark and Fletcher 1999)

Practical considerations

- Will the mattress fit on the patient's existing bed? Consider both the width and the change in height. Does the patient share a double bed with his or her partner?
- How easy is the support surface to transport and to set up?

- Will staff need to be trained to use the equipment and will staff be required to supervise its use? This is particularly important if it is to be used in the patient's home.
- How should it be cleaned in between patient use and how much storage space does it require? How much maintenance is required and who will perform this?
- Is the patient within the correct weight/height limit suggested by the manufacturer?
- Is the mattress acceptable to the patient? (Clark and Fletcher 1999)

Financial considerations

Financial factors often affect the availability of support surfaces to patients. The following points need to be considered to avoid incurring unnecessary costs and to allow equity of access to equipment.

- Is there a clear procedure for 'stepping up and down' to ensure that equipment is removed from patients who no longer need that level of equipment, so that other more needy individuals can gain access to it?
- Are there any hidden costs, e.g. maintenance costs or specialist cleaning?
- What will it cost the patient or relatives to run the equipment, and is this acceptable to them?

Q9.9   What type of support surface should be selected?

There is a large selection of support surfaces available. They can be divided into those providing pressure reduction and those providing pressure relief. Pressure reduction is the constant relief of pressure that is being exerted on the patient's body. This is produced by equipment such as layered or formed foam-, gel-, fibre- or air-filled mattresses, low air-loss or air-fluidised systems (Kenney and Rithalia 1999).

Pressure relief is intermittent lowering of the external pressure on the patient's body by inflation and deflation of the cells of the mattress or by lifting the body clear of the surface. This can be achieved by manual turns, or by the use of an alternating pressure mattress.

Static overlays are the simplest form of pressure-reducing mattresses (Collier 1999a). They can be made of foam, fibre or gel, which conforms to the patient's body shape and redistributes weight over a larger surface area.

There are a number of static mattresses with pressure-reducing properties available. These are made of foam. Consideration should be given to the density and the hardness of the foam, higher density foam usually lasting longer than low-density foam (Kenney and Rithalia 1999). The mattress may be designed with foam slits or be preformed to fit the patient's contours. All these mattresses are designed to distribute pressure evenly under the patient. Consideration should be given to how often the mattress needs turning to keep it in good condition, and what type of fabric the cover is made of (Collier 1999a). Static cushions are available and should have the same qualities as the mattress chosen.

Low air-loss systems are available either as bed systems or mattresses and provide pressure reduction via individual air-filled cells, often grouped regionally to maximise the pressure-reducing effect.

Alternating pressure surfaces can be supplied as overlays or replacement mattresses. They consist of a number of sealed cells in a removable cover, which inflate and deflate alternately, thus redistributing the pressure over the soft tissues of the body and allowing reperfusion of previously supported areas (McLeod 1997).

Natural sheepskins may reduce friction or shear but do not reduce pressure (Collier 1999b). Synthetic sheepskins have been shown to be ineffective and, if poorly laundered, to increase interface pressure (Lothian and Barbenal 1983).

Rubber or Sorbo rings should never be used to reduce pressure, because they actually concentrate pressure on a smaller surface and may cause new ulcers (Lothian and Barbenal 1983).

Suggestions for types of mattress are difficult. Ideally, all health-care areas should have a local policy that suggests equipment based on clinical effectiveness. The *Effective Health Care Bulletin* (1995) states that 'most of the equipment available for the prevention and treatment of pressure sores has not been reliably evaluated and no "best buy" can be recommended'.

A general guide could be the following:

- Grade 1/2 sore: static overlay/cushion
- Grade 2/3 sore: alternating airwave overlay/cushion
- Grade 3/4 sore: alternating airwave mattress/cushion.

However, a patient with no sore may indicate a high level of risk and require an appropriate support surface. Immobile patients who cannot turn will need regular position changes to keep them free of sores.

Summary

Pressure sores are caused by extrinsic and intrinsic factors. The risk of damage developing should be predicted using a suitable, reliable and valid tool. Pressure damage should be prevented by both selecting an appropriate support surface and alleviating the effects of the intrinsic factors that contribute to pressure damage.

CHAPTER 10

Wound infection

This chapter discusses the care of infected wounds, how to recognise wound infection and how it should be treated. The principles of cross-infections and asepsis are addressed and the precautions that are necessary to deal with patients who have MRSA.

For further information about infection control the reader is referred to Duggal, Beaumont and Jenkinson, *Infection Control: A Handbook for Community Nurses* – in this series.

Q10.1 How is wound infection recognised?

Infected tissue within a wound often has a greenish appearance. Routine swabbing of wounds is inappropriate for diagnosis of infection and an unnecessary cost (see Q10.3). It is important to understand that wounds may have transient organisms present, which swab results detect in small numbers. These organisms are often the usual skin flora and are not usually regarded as pathogenic.

Many chronic wounds become colonised by a variety of bacteria which may be potentially pathogenic. Colonisation means that the organisms have multiplied and are often present in large numbers, although infection is not inevitable and many colonised wounds heal without problem. These micro-organisms can, however, be dispersed during dressing changes and measures should be taken to limit this.

Wound infection occurs when colonising bacteria reach sufficient numbers to cause distinct clinical signs (Table 10.1).

If a wound exhibits one or more of these signs, it is appropriate to take a wound swab. Patients who are immunocompromised or diabetic may fail to show signs of inflammation and signs of clinical infection, and may require a swab to be taken if the wound is failing

Table 10.1 Signs of wound infection

Erythema
Oedema
Increased exudate
Offensive odour
Pain
Pyrexia
(Thompson and Smith 1994)

to respond to treatment, even if the usual clinical signs are not present. Occasionally, other patients may not exhibit the classic immune response (Plewa 1990). If wounds are failing to respond to treatment, it is worth considering the following seven other criteria (Table 10.2) that may indicate infection, suggested by Cutting and Harding (1994).

Table 10.2 Other indications of wound infection

Delayed healing
Discoloration
Friable granulation tissue which bleeds easily
Unexpected tenderness
Pocketing at the base of the wound
Bridging of soft tissue and epithelium
Wound breakdown
(Cutting and Harding 1994)

Q10.2 What factors increase the chances of wound infection occurring?

The chance of wound infection will increase with the length of hospital stay, with very young and very elderly patients being more prone to infection, plus patients who are immunosuppressed, have diabetes (see Q8.18) or are malnourished (see Q3.4), and where the patient interferes with their wound. The following two scenarios illustrate this.

Case study 7

Mrs J was an articulate and well-dressed woman of 60 who had self-cared for her leg ulcer for several years before she was referred to the practice nurse. A full assessment, including Doppler studies, indicated that the ulcer was of venous origin. Treatment was commenced with a foam dressing and single-layer compression, and the treatment was to be changed once a week.

Initially the ulcer responded well and was reducing in size. After a few weeks it became infected and needed treatment with antibiotics. The infection resolved. After another couple of weeks the ulcer again became infected and antibiotics were required. This became a pattern over the next couple of months and no progress towards healing was being made. Eventually, after gentle questioning, it was revealed that Mrs J wanted her leg dressed more frequently than once a week as she had always done it once or twice a day when looking after it herself. To achieve this she was taking off the bandage, washing and drying the foam dressing and carefully rebandaging the limb. The nurse explained to her that this was the cause of the frequent infections and that it was preferable that the dressing be left in place to optimise wound healing.

To achieve a better level of compliance, a compromise was reached whereby she attended the surgery twice a week. The ulcer again started to progress and finally went on to heal.

Case study 8

Mr H was a 76-year-old farmer. He had always been active and still managed a small mixed farm including cows, ducks, sheep and hens. He had recently developed a venous leg ulcer which had developed rapidly and kept getting infected. This situation was not helped by copious amounts of farmyard manure. His condition was starting to limit his mobility and his ability to take care of the farm. This was making him extremely anxious. Two-layer compression bandaging had been attempted, but constant pulling off of Wellington boots kept disturbing the bandages which were filthy with manure.

A four-layer bandage had been considered but, with the amount of exudate and the necessity for the Wellington boot, dismissed. After a joint consultation of the vascular specialist, tissue viability nurse, district nurse, Mr H and his sister, it was agreed that the priorities were to reduce the amount of infection and thereby the exudate, and to achieve a good level of compression. Four-layer bandaging was commenced, Mr H's sister purchased a larger Wellington boot and cut it down to half leg length to aid easier application and removal, and a pop sock over the bandage made it less sticky, which also helped. Initially the bandage was changed twice a week.

Mr H's legs improved dramatically, the exudate decreased, the bandages stayed in place and the farmyard manure did not penetrate the layers of bandage, and so the infections subsided. His mobility returned. After 6 months of treatment, the leg was healed and Mr H continued to run his farm.

Q10.3 Is there a recommended method of taking a wound swab?

There is some controversy over the best method of performing a wound swab. The method described by Cooper and Lawrence (1996) is gently to irrigate the wound with physiological saline, to use the swab in a zig-zag motion over the entire wound surface while slowly rotating it.

Q10.4 How should infected wounds be treated?

Treatment of infection should be with systemic antibiotics, because the use of topical treatments with antibacterial creams can lead to the growth of resistant organisms, and should be avoided (Morgan 1987).

Untreated wound infection can lead to septicaemia and death (see Q10.13).

Q10.5 What is cellulitis and how should it be treated?

Cellulitis is an acute, rapidly swelling inflammation of the skin and soft tissues (Grey 1998). It is characterised by swelling, pain, erythema and heat, and sometimes fever. These signs are usually confined to the area around the wound, but in some severe cases it may be accompanied by features of systemic toxicity, including septicaemia. It often occurs after minor breaks in the skin, lacerations, surgical wounds and ulcers.

The two main causative organisms are *Staphylococcus aureus* and *Streptococcus pyogenes* (Grey 1998). Streptococcal infection tends to be associated with small breaks in the skin and staphylococcal infections with larger wounds such as ulcers.

Identification of the causative organism is often difficult, with tests such as wound swabs and blood cultures giving poor results. Diagnosis and treatment tend to be empirical and based on the bacteriology of the associated wound. However, culture of any tissue fluid or pus should be attempted. Blood should be taken if there are clinical signs of infection, but these tests are not always positive even if there are signs of systemic infection (Grey 1998). Severe cases will require hospital admission.

Patients with diabetic or ischaemic foot ulcers (see Q8.18), who develop associated cellulitis, are at high risk of developing systemic toxicity (Grey 1998), and if undertreated this can have grave consequences such as the loss of a limb.

Treatment is normally a systemic antibiotic (Morison and Moffatt 1994); infection present within the tissues cannot be reached by applying topical agents (see Q10.4).

> Q10.6 What is the single most important thing that can be done in clinical practice to reduce the risk of cross-infection?

Effective hand washing is the most important factor in reducing cross-infection (Parker 1999). Although this is routinely acknowledged, a constant application of this practice still does not exist. Micro-organisms found on the skin are termed 'resident' and 'transient' flora.

'Resident' organisms live and multiply on the skin and will vary from person to person. They generally are not virulent and rarely cause the person harm. However, if transferred to deeper structures they could be harmful, e.g. during invasive procedures such as minor surgery. Hazard can be minimised by using an antiseptic hand wash (Parker 1999.)

'Transient' organisms are acquired from contact with another person or object, such as from contaminated surfaces. During 'dirty' procedures, e.g. changing the dressing on an infected wound, they can be picked up even when gloves are worn. They tend to be loosely attached, so washing with soap and water will remove them.

Hands should be washed as follows:

1. Rub palm to palm
2. Rub backs of both hands

3. Rub palms again with fingers interlaced
4. Rub backs of interlaced fingers
5. Remember to wash both thumbs
6. Rub both palms with finger tips.

Washing should be under running water with chosen cleanser and hands should be thoroughly dried on a paper towel. Routine social hand washing should be 10–15 seconds with either soap or an antiseptic, whereas for minor surgery washing should be 2–5 minutes.

Other points to consider are:

1. Avoid wearing jewellery especially rings (wedding rings should be manipulated during hand washing to remove micro-organisms).
2. Keep nails short.
3. Wet hands before applying handwash agent.
4. Use only non-ionic handcream; do not use communal jars.
5. Always cover any cuts with a waterproof dressing.
6. Handwash agents can become contaminated; bar soap should be allowed to drain dry (no slimy soap dishes); do not top up liquid soap or antiseptic agents.
7. If hands show signs of irritation get medical advice (Parker 1999).

Q10.7 What is MRSA?

MRSA stands for methicillin (or multi)-resistant *Staphylococcus aureus*. *Staphylococcus aureus* is a bacteria carried by 20–40% of the population with no ill effects (Weaver 1996); it colonises the skin, nasal passages and mouth.

Widespread use of antibiotics has led to an emergence of resistant strains. MRSA is resistant to penicillin, important anti-staphylococcal agents such as flucloxacillin, cephalosporins and other related antibiotics.

If a patient has a severe clinical infection of MRSA, he or she will need hospitalisation and treatment with intravenous vancomycin, but most patients are colonised rather than infected.

If the patient is a heavy carrier and disperser, although not at risk to him- or herself other patients who are sick or have wounds may be at risk from cross-infection (Wolverhampton Health Care Control of Infection Committee 1995).

Q10.8 What swabs should be taken to screen for MRSA?

Swabs should be pre-moistened with sterile saline in order to collect more bacteria. The following sites are recommended:

- External nares (nostrils)
- Axilla and groin
- Any wounds
- Sputum (if the patient has a productive cough)
- The wound itself
- If the patient has a catheter, a urine specimen.

A patient is clear when three sets of swabs at weekly intervals are negative after any treatment is terminated.

Q10.9 How should a patient who is a carrier of MRSA be treated?

The patient should be advised to have a daily bath or strip wash. He or she should apply an antiseptic detergent directly to the skin with a wash cloth and rinse off. If the axilla and groin are colonised, hexachlorophene powder should be applied.

Hair should be washed daily and on the first and third day of treatment washed with an antiseptic detergent. After bathing the patient should put on clean clothes. Bed linen should be changed as frequently as possible. Laundry can go on a normal wash preferably at 60°C. If the external nares are colonised, mupirocin ointment is applied three times a day for 7 days.

The patient poses no risk to anyone in his or her own home unless they have a wound, catheter or other invasive line (Weaver 1996). Visitors should be advised that they are at no special risk and that excessive hand washing with antiseptics may make the patient feel isolated. It is recommended that antiseptic hand washing is beneficial only if there is prolonged contact or dirty materials such as dressings have been handled. This is not the case for visiting nurses or home helps who may be in contact with other at-risk individuals afterwards (see Q10.10).

The patient can continue with normal social activities. There are no restrictions on using public transport. If the patient needs to go to outpatients, ambulance control should be informed, as should the outpatients department. If the patient requires hospital admission the receiving doctor should be informed.

General domestic cleaning is adequate, although it is important to keep the environment as clean as possible, especially dust control. Any home carers/home helps should be educated in good hand-washing techniques and have disposable gloves and aprons available. If the patient has equipment on loan such as mattresses or commodes, the loan centre should be informed before the return of any equipment.

Q10.10 What precautions should the district nurse take?

District nurses should use disposable gloves and aprons, which can then be disposed of in the patient's normal household waste (Wolverhampton Health Care Control of Infection Committee 1995). Hands should be washed thoroughly with antiseptic handwash such as Hibiscub. Paper towels should be left in the house for use rather than using household towels. Any cuts or abrasions should be covered with a waterproof plaster (Weaver 1996).

Patients infected or colonised with MRSA should have their dressings changed at the end of the day. Rubbish should be disposed of in line with the local infection control policy.

When the patient no longer requires dressings no left-over stocks should be taken out of the house for use in other areas.

Q10.11 What precautions should be taken in the GP surgery for a patient with MRSA infection?

Patients who are MRSA positive or awaiting swab results should have their dressings attended to at the end of the day's surgery. The wound should be cleaned with a chlorhexidine-based solution. If the patient has flaky skin, such as those with venous eczema, care should be taken to catch all skin flakes.

Staff members are at no personal risk because the MRSA does not pose a risk to healthy individuals (Weaver 1996).

Good hand-washing technique is the best method of controlling spread of MRSA and the use of gloves (in line with your local infection control policy) and aprons is recommended (Duckworth 1990).

Hands should be washed with an antiseptic chlorhexidine agent or with an alcohol rub, and dried on disposable paper towels. Any open cuts should be covered with a waterproof plaster.

All soiled dressings should be bagged and sealed in infected waste bags and sent for incineration, in line with your local infection control policy; contact your local infection control nurse for advice.

Q10.12 Are there any specific guidelines for nursing/residential homes?

Patients should be cared for in a single room and away from other patients with open wounds or breaks in the skin (Wolverhampton Health Care Control of Infection Committee 1995). Ensuite hand-washing facilities should be available if possible and an antiseptic hand wash available. The patient's personal clothing and bed linen should be cared for as infected in accordance with the home's policy. Contact your local infection control department to see if there is a specific 'Nursing Home' policy. General cleaning with a general purpose detergent is satisfactory. Damp dusting is recommended.

Q10.13 What is the recommended management for wounds colonised with MRSA?

Topical antibiotics are often advocated for the treatment of MRSA. There is, however, concern about the efficacy if they are applied infrequently or over a large area (Weaver 1996) (see Q10.4).

Two antibiotics are recommended and treatment should be no longer than 7–14 days. Mupirocin can be applied to shallow wounds no larger than 3 cm in diameter. Fusidic acid is a good anti-staphylococcal agent but, if used alone or over a large area, resistance may occur. It may be useful in combination with oral trimethoprim for 10 days.

After the antibiotics have stopped, the wound should be treated according to its clinical appearance, e.g. sloughy, necrotic, etc. Two days after antibiotic therapy has stopped, repeat wound swabs should be taken. If the wound is colonised or not severely infected, it may respond to antiseptics alone. Dressings such as Flamazine and Inadine have been found to be effective against some strains of MRSA.

Q10.14 Do staff need to be screened for MRSA?

MRSA does not pose a threat to staff. Therefore a staff member caring for a patient with MRSA is at no personal risk, nor are their families. Becoming a carrier of MRSA is no reflection on an individual's personal hygiene.

If infection control precautions are taken the risk of becoming a carrier is minimal. However, in an institution where several patients are MRSA positive, it is possible that staff may become carriers (Wolverhampton Health Care Control of Infection Committee 1995). If staff do become carriers they can easily be treated with antiseptic preparations. Staff can be screened with agreement with the local infection control team and they or the occupational health department will advise on treatment and when to return to work.

Summary

Routine swabbing is ineffective and an unnecessary waste of money. It important to recognise signs of infection. Wound infection should be treated systemically. Be aware of the principles of cross-infection and asepsis. Also be aware of necessary precautions if the patient has MRSA.

CHAPTER 11

Miscellaneous

This chapter deals with other frequently asked questions that do not fit into any of the other chapters in the book. These include care of fungating wounds, dressing difficult areas, maceration and the use of maggots (larval therapy).

> Q11.1 What is a fungating wound?

Fungating describes a condition of ulceration and proliferation that arises when malignant tumour cells infiltrate and erode through the skin (Mortimer 1993), or malignant cells spread along pathways of least resistance, e.g. between tissue planes and lymph capillaries (Mosely 1988). Fungating tumours may be complicated by sinus or fistula formation.

Fungating tumours develop in a number of sites. Most common is the breast but melanoma, lymphoma, and cancers of the lung, stomach, head, neck, uterus, kidney, ovary, colon and bladder may also infiltrate in this way (Mortimer 1993).

Tissue hypoxia in a fungating wound is a significant problem leading to a loss of tissue viability. Anaerobic and aerobic bacteria thrive in these conditions and are the cause of the associated malodour and profuse exudate (Groscott 1995). In addition, the capillaries of tumours are fragile and predispose the tissue to bleeding. Tumour growth results in wounds that are continually enlarging, irregular in shape, necrotic and exuding.

Wound management is complex and involves managing odour (see Q2.6), exudate (see Q5.2), bleeding (see Q11.2) and pain control (see Q2.7–Q2.9).

105

Q11.2 How can bleeding in fragile fungating wounds be controlled?

Capillary bleeding can occur for a number of reasons. As tumours enlarge the blood vessels become eroded and blood loss can cause anaemia (Dealey 1994). Inappropriate removal of a dressing causes clots to loosen. Alginates have haemostatic properties that are valuable in the control of bleeding (see Q5.9). The concentration of calcium ions in the alginate facilitates the exchange with sodium ions in the wound exudate, activating the clotting mechanism and forming a viscous gel. Alginate dressings can be removed with gentle irrigation, further reducing capillary trauma.

To control profuse bleeding, occasionally cautery or oral anti-fibrinolytic agents are used (Thomas and Vowden 1998). Topical adrenaline should only ever be used with caution and under medical supervision (Dealey 1994). Emflorgo (1998) advocates mixing sucralfate with a water-soluble gel and applying this as a primary dressing covered by a low adherent dressing.

Q11.3 Can aromatherapy oils be used in the treatment of chronic wounds?

In recent years interest in complementary therapies has been increasing in both the general public and health-care workers.

Oils specifically mentioned in relation to topical application to assist wound healing are tea tree oil and lavender oil. However, it is an area that needs further research, because most currently available evidence is anecdotal (Asquith 1999).

It should be remembered that, although the practice of aromatherapy has many benefits, essential oils are powerful chemicals with risks attached to their use, and they should be used only by a qualified aromatherapist (Asquith 1999). If they are to be used as a 'topical medication', they should really be pharmacologically tested as any other topical medication would be.

Q11.4 Some wounds such as those on fingers or elbows can be difficult to
        dress. Any tips for application?

Areas that commonly cause difficulties include areas over joints where there is a problem retaining mobility without loss of integrity of the dressing, especially digits where it can be difficult to apply and retain a dressing while allowing normal functioning, and heels where the dressing has to be shaped (Fletcher 1999). To dress heels, a flat dressing such as a hydrocolloid or foam can be cut and then shaped around the heel.

To dress digits, many people use a cotton net and applicator to secure the primary dressing. Other solutions include cutting a flat product to allow it to be shaped around the digit without too much bulk. If the dressing requires securing with tape, ensure that the tape does not completely wrap around the finger. If oedema occurs it could cause constriction.

Dressings over joints such as elbows or the knee can restrict mobility because the dressing does not stretch or it is bulky. Cutting a thin hydrocolloid or film and applying it in slightly overlapping strips will allow some flexibility (Fletcher 1999). This can be used either as a primary dressing or a retention dressing. Usually no other bulky padding is required.

Q11.5 What causes skin maceration?

Maceration is caused by prolonged exposure to fluid that remains in contact with the skin. This may be wound exudate, urine or sweat. It may cause deterioration in the wound and also lead to skin breakdown.

The body's normal wound-healing response of inflammation causes local oedema, which seeps from the wound surface (see Q1.8). The exudate from acute and chronic wounds has different constituents (Cutting 1999). The exudate from chronic wounds contains proteases, which break down protein and will actually damage what may be otherwise healthy tissue (Hofman et al. 1997). Exudate production often increases if the wound deteriorates.

Moist wound healing has been shown to speed up wound healing (Winter 1962) (see Q1.9) and many dressings such as films, foams, hydrocolloids, alginates and hydrofibres promote healing using the theory of moist wound healing (see Q5.2).

Occlusive dressings (see Q5.6) are often blamed for maceration (Cutting 1999) but it will only occur if the dressing regimen is being used inappropriately. Wear time should not exceed the time beyond which the dressing can adequately cope with the production of exudate. The choice of dressing needs to reflect exudate levels as well as the site and condition of the wound. Hydrofibre and alginate dressings are very absorbent and can be covered with absorbent pads (see Q5.9 and Q5.14).

Exudate from venous ulcers can be controlled with compression therapy and elevation when clinically indicated (Cutting 1999) (see Q8.29).

If skin becomes macerated, some people use eosin as an astringent to dry it (do not use on the actual wound) (Morgan 1997). Others soak the leg, including the wound, in a solution of potassium permanganate. Neither of these two approaches has been evaluated in comparative clinical trials (Cutting 1999).

Zinc oxide paste or bandages may be used to provide protection by acting as a barrier. It is worth patch testing before full application to avoid sensitivity. If high levels of exudate persist, the possibility of infection should be considered. (see Q10.1 and Q10.2).

Q11.6 What is meant by overgranulation and how should I treat it?

Overgranulation, or hypergranulation as it is sometimes called, is granulation tissue that rises above the edges of the wound. Experience has shown that removing an interactive dressing such as a hydrocolloid and using a simple dressing such as a low adherent dressing or foam allows the wound to settle down on its own. Silver nitrate used either as a 0.25% compress or as a silver nitrate stick is also sometimes used (Morgan 1997).

The use of maggots: larval therapy

Q11.7 Are maggots available only for treating wounds in hospital?

There is no reason why maggots or larvae cannot be used for patients within their own homes or a nursing home, providing that the patient and their family are in agreement. However, larvae are not on prescription at present and so funding would have to be provided by the primary care group or trust.

Q11.8 What types of wound are suitable for treatment with larvae?

Maggots remove both dead tissue and bacteria, leaving in most cases a healthy granulating wound (Thomas et al. 1996). Their main use would be on a necrotic, sloughy or infected wound (see Q2.10 and Q2.11 and Tables 10.1 and 10.2).

Q11.9 How are the maggots applied to the wound?

The most common method of application is to surround the wound with a border of hydrocolloid. This is applied to the intact skin like a picture frame. The maggots are flushed out of their carriage containers with saline and applied to the wound surface, approximately 10 larvae/cm^2 (Thomas et al. 1996.) Maggots are approximately 2 mm in length. A piece of sterile, fine nylon mesh covers the maggots and wound, and is held in position by sticking it to the hydrocolloid with adhesive tape. Gauze dampened with physiological saline is placed over this to keep the maggots hydrated. Any padding can then be applied to contain exudate and liquefied necrotic tissue. The maggots should be changed every 3–4 days.

Q11.10 How should maggots be removed and disposed of?

When the soiled dressings are removed the larvae either fall off or can be flushed off the wound surface with saline. Dressings should be placed in a yellow bag, sealed securely and sent for incineration.

Q11.11 Is there any risk of maggots turning into flies?

A newly hatched larvae takes 7–14 days to complete its life cycle and turn into a fly. As dressings are changed every 3–4 days they will be removed from the wound well before they pupate and turn into a fly.

Q11.12 Can the patient feel the maggots moving on the wound or eating the dead tissue?

Most patients cannot feel the maggots on the wound. If they are on intact skin they may tickle but surrounding the wound with hydrocolloid eliminates this.

The majority of patients receiving larval therapy report a reduction in wound-related pain (Thomas et al. 1996), although a few report an increase in pain (see Q2.7–Q2.9). The sterile larvae supplied do not burrow into healthy tissue.

Information

Q11.13 Are there any sources of information about wound care on the internet?

There are many sources of information about wound care on the internet. General search engines can be used as well as tools to assist in locating medical information and direct access uniform resource locators (URLs) to appropriate sites.

This is becoming an increasingly popular way of searching the literature. Information is accessible worldwide at any time and to anyone with the appropriate technology. It is a rich educational source which can assist educational development; it also gives an e-mail link with research foundations and other contributors and thus aids the easy discussion of findings (Pitcher 1998).

Some useful web sites are listed under Resources, pp. 134–5.

Summary

Fungating wounds can be complex to treat, and specialist advice may be needed. The need for sensitive care when dealing with malodorous wounds cannot be overstressed. Maggots can be a useful and effective therapy, which is currently gaining in popularity. Patient education and support are essential for compliance with this therapy.

CHAPTER 12

Clinical effectiveness

Clinical effectiveness is about ensuring that we provide the best possible care, in the right environment, at the optimum time, and in a sensitive and effective manner. It brings together patients' wants and needs, with the nurses' expertise from training and experience, and the best available research evidence to provide the highest quality patient care.

This chapter explores both what clinical effectiveness is, and the skills and processes involved. Sources of evidence and information, and their use in everyday practice, are discussed. Approaches are drawn not only from research evidence, but also from patients' views and experiences at both individual and group levels. A variety of tools is discussed, including clinical audit, patient interviews, focus groups, reflective practice and critical incidents or significant event analysis. These tools can help the nurse be confident of providing the best possible service, and can give the satisfaction of continuously maintaining and developing her or his skills.

> Q12.1 How can the nurse ensure that the best possible care is provided for the patient?

There is a variety of techniques that can be used; these are examined in a little more depth. Tools and resources that you can access include clinical audit and effectiveness, comments and complaints, investigating patient experiences, critical incidence analysis and reflective practice. This chapter explores these tools, and how they can be used to provide clinically effective and patient-friendly care.

Q12.2 What is clinical effectiveness?

Clinical effectiveness or evidence-based health care is an approach to practice that helps you to consider whether you are providing optimum care for your patients through identifying existing evidence on best practice. The chart shown in Figure 12.1 was produced by the North Thames Research Appraisal Group (1998) to help guide people in ensuring that they are making the best possible use of research in their clinical practice.

There are several steps to developing the process and skills involved in ensuring that the care you provide is evidence based. You may feel that you currently do not possess all of the skills that are involved in the process, and if this is the case do not worry, we all have a lot to learn. There are lots of people who can lend their skills and expertise to help you along the way. Addressing the stages of the process in a little more depth will identify who the key people are to contact for help in developing your expertise in this area. You might find it helpful to raise any training needs that you identify at your next performance review meeting.

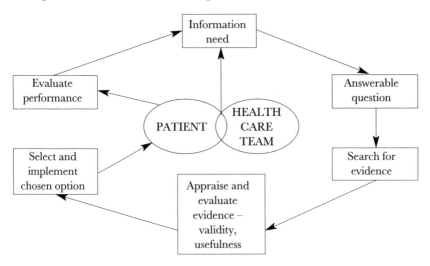

Figure 12.1 The clinical effectiveness process.

Q12.3 What information is needed?

This question is really asking about where the gaps in the management of your patients are. Each patient is unique and may come with one hundred and one different questions, so you will almost always find that there is something for you to discover. Questions can be about all aspects of patient care. In wound care they may include things such as:

- What is the best sort of dressing for this wound?
- How long will it take to heal?
- Would physiotherapy help?
- How can I stop another ulcer developing?

Once you start thinking about issues regarding all your different patients, you will probably find that you have far more potential questions than you could possibly find the time to answer so you will need to decide what the key problems are and how to prioritise. Topics that are likely to come to the top of the priority list include problems common to a number of patients, unusually severe or serious presentations of conditions, concerns about the quality of the service raised by staff, patients or relatives, and areas where there is perceived to be real potential to improve the quality of care.

Q12.4 What does it mean to ask an answerable question?

Once you have thought about the issues and concerns that are of interest to you, it is worth formulating them into a clear question. This will help you to target your search for the answer to the question. These questions tend to include four elements:

- The key features of the patient or problem.
- Details of the intervention or test that you are considering.
- Possible alternatives to that intervention.
- Indications of the outcomes of interest.

When identifying the key features of the patient or problem you should think about how you would describe a similar group of patients. This may include aspects such as condition, age, sex and ethnicity. The intervention or test and possible alternatives refer to what you think your options are in treating your patients. You may have to decide between two different types of bandages or dressing, or answer more general questions about what is the best form of footwear for someone who has foot ulceration when you are not yet aware of the possible options. Outcomes can come from a variety of perspectives, whether that of the patient, carers, doctors or nursing staff, and on occasion can conflict with each other. Your main aim may be the complete healing of a wound, whereas the patient may be desperate to maintain mobility and independence, and so may be prepared to accept continuing ulceration in return for that freedom.

To help put this into some sort of context, a short scenario can show how that can be used to devise an answerable question.

The scenario

When people come to see you about wound care, you currently give them verbal advice about treating the wound, diet, exercise and lifestyle. You have recently developed several concerns about this. You have read that generally people only remember 10% of what they have been told during consultations and are particularly concerned that a substantial number of the local population belong to ethnic minority groups and do not speak English as their first language. You have therefore decided to review the way you provide information to your patients.

The question

Element	Example
Patient or problem	People with wounds who do not speak English as their first language
Intervention or test	Simple verbal explanation supported by written material (possibly in relevant languages)
Possible alternatives	Cassettes and video tapes in relevant languages, accessing interpretation services
Outcome(s) of interest	Understanding and retention of information, compliance with recommendations, increased healing rates for wounds

Your question is therefore likely to be something like:

Is it more effective to provide oral, written, cassette or video advice for people with wound care needs who do not speak English as their first language in order to ensure that they understand and remember the advice, comply with treatment and have wounds that heal?

Q12.5 How do I search for evidence?

The first port of call for most of us when we have a clinical question is to consult a colleague. This is an entirely legitimate action and the professional knowledge that you and your colleagues share is a key factor in patient care. However, you also need to be aware that it is impossible for anyone to stay abreast of current practice and research in all areas of care. Reading all the journal articles that come out each month about community nursing would in itself be more than a full-time job, and you are still expected to keep seeing the patients! Like your colleagues, textbooks can become rapidly out of date, and in some areas of medicine it is estimated that the textbooks will be out of date before they even hit the shelves, so you will need to turn to other sources of evidence and make friends with your local librarian who can assist you in this.

The best evidence that you can find comes when comprehensive literature searches have been done to answer questions about specific areas of care, the results considered for their quality and then combined to indicate best possible practice in the given area. This is known as a systematic review or meta-analysis. These can be used to produce guidelines on best practice. An example of this is the *Effective Health Care Bulletins* produced by the Centre for Reviews and Dissemination at York University. Topics covered include prevention and treatment of pressure sores and management of venous ulcers, and copies of these should be available through your practice, clinic or your local librarian or local audit adviser. Other sources are databases of systemic reviews including the Cochrane Library, Database of Reviews of Effectiveness and Best Evidence, and your local librarian should be able to put you in touch with these. It is also worth contacting the Royal College of Nursing and other professional bodies to see whether they have produced evidence-based guidelines.

If you cannot find the answer to your question in a systematic review or through your professional body, you will need to undertake your own literature search. There are various databases that you can search. The main ones that you are likely to come across are Medline, which includes abstracts and details of articles produced in over 1000 different medical and related journals worldwide, and CINAHL (Cumulative Index of Nursing and Allied Health Literature) which again contains abstracts and details of articles in nursing and professional clinical service journals. Again your librarian should be able to advise you how to be able to tap into these resources effectively.

One of the main sources you can use to search for information is via the internet. One of the issues raised by the case study on providing information relates to a possible need for written information for patients. If your literature search indicated that this would be effective then you could also search for user disease-based groups who may already be providing information, which you could integrate with the resources that you provide for your patients. Many of these groups now have websites on the internet (see Q11.13).

Q12.6 How can I learn to appraise evidence?

Clinical appraisal is a technique to assist you in reviewing research to ensure that the results are valid, believable, impressive and applicable. Checklists have been produced for different types of research such as qualitative trials comparing different interventions (randomised controlled trials or RCTs), trials looking at the pattern of an illness or disease over time (longitudinal studies), etc. by organisations such as NTRAG (North Thames Research Appraisal Group) and CASP (Critical Appraisal Skills Programme). The clinical governance lead of your primary care group or trust should be able to arrange for you to have some training on this either through local training initiatives or CD ROM-based learning packs which may be available within the organisation.

In order to develop your skills in this area, it would be worth considering joining a journal club. Journal clubs consist of small groups of staff who meet regularly to discuss research papers and their application to practice. If you don't feel like joining one with GPs you could think about setting one up with other practice staff.

Q12.7 So if I go through all this process, identify my problem, find some evidence that helps answer it and introduce some changes to my practice, how do I know whether or not it has had the desired effect?

This is where the next stage of the clinical effectiveness process comes in as you can start to think about evaluating your performance, reflecting on what has worked well and what needs to be changed to be even more effective. Tools that can be useful in this process include clinical audit, patient participation and reflective practice.

Q12.8 What is clinical audit?

Clinical audit is a tool to help you reflect on your clinical practice and to evaluate the effectiveness of the care that you provide (Figure 12.2).

As in the clinical effectiveness process you need to identify the area or issue of concern and seek to identify what current best practice is in this area. You use this to set standards for the care process. For wound care these could include:

- All patients presenting with leg ulcers have a thorough assessment including Doppler studies.
- All patients with venous ulcers receive compression therapy.
- All patients are provided with written information about the care and management of venous ulcers and related health and lifestyle advice.

Having set your standards, you then need to decide the best way of identifying whether they have been achieved. This can be through a variety of techniques including reviewing patient notes, downloading information from the practice computer and collecting specific

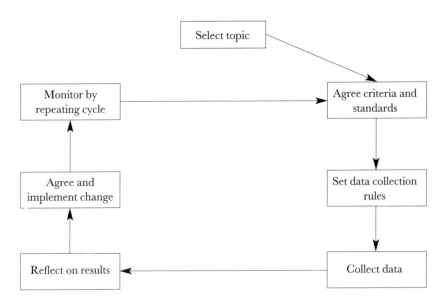

Figure 12.2 The clinical audit cycle.

information over a limited time scale. Your practice, clinic, or primary care group or trust may be lucky enough to have an information technology (IT) or computer specialist who could advise you on retrieving information from information systems.

For the standards listed above, you may decide to create a checklist which you could use while going through the notes to tick off whether or not each standard has been achieved. You may wish to add a comments column in which you can record such things as gaps in the patient history or length of time since the last Doppler result was recorded if it was not in the previous 3 months.

It is very hard to look objectively at our own notes and practice, so you might find it helpful to join up with some other practice nurses or community staff and agree to look at each other's notes. Coming to a set of notes with fresh eyes, you often notice things that you would overlook in your own notes, and you can learn from other people's good practice and their mistakes. You could also learn whether your hand-writing is likely to be legible for someone covering you when you are on holiday or for someone taking over if you should choose to change jobs.

If you are reviewing patient records, you will need to decide how many notes to select to provide a representative sample. If you pull only one set of notes you might find that the results are exceptionally poor or good, but you would not know whether the results for that patient were abnormal for some reason. Books on statistics provide sampling tables that you could use to decide how many notes you would need to review to be confident that the results were not the result of chance. These are based on the population size, i.e. the number of people with the particular condition that you are looking at, not the population of the entire practice. However, you may feel that, rather than pursue a rigid statistical approach, you would be happy to get a feel of what is happening in your practice. In this case you may choose to select the last 10 sets of notes of people you saw with the chosen problem or select one set for each of the first letters in the alphabet. This approach is also helpful when you are keen to review your practice but have only very limited time to devote to it. In such circumstances, providing you are prepared to take on board the results whether they are good or bad, you can legitimately review smaller numbers of notes.

Once you have collected your data, you need to think about compiling the results and developing an action plan. You will probably find that there are some areas where you have performed to a very high standard and others where there is room for improvement. You will then need to develop an action plan to identify what you are going to do about the areas of concern that have been highlighted. This might include things that you can do immediately such as ensuring that you take and record a Doppler reading on a regular basis (see Q8.12) and outcomes that would take longer to achieve, such as obtaining or producing appropriate literature on different sorts of wounds to provide to patients. If tasks cannot be done immediately, set yourself a deadline for achieving each area and put these in your diary, as well as in your action plan to help ensure that they will happen. You may find things that are out of your control, such as a need for dressings that are not available in the primary care group (PCG) formulary. You could share the results of the audit with the practice team to help inform the debate about resource allocation, to provide the best possible care for your patient population within the available resources. Even when there are no resource implications, it is a good idea to share what you have done with your peers and colleagues. You deserve recognition both for undertaking the audit and for the good practice you have identified, and in reporting your proposed improvements you are committing yourself to making change where there is room for improvement.

The last thing that you need to put on your action plan is your reaudit date. When you have gone through the process and made some changes, you need to review your practice again to ensure that the changes have had the desired results and that the improvements in patient care have been sustained. This may be done by repeating the whole audit, by looking at a smaller number of cases or by concentrating on areas where problems were identified during the original survey.

Case note reviews and review of practice-held data are just a couple of the ways of reflecting on the quality of the care that you provide. Your standards may include some more intangible areas of care such as patients feeling that they have been treated with dignity and respect, provision of information and the maintenance of confidentiality, which you cannot measure from written notes or other documentation. You may find you need to review the waiting room to see whether posters provide appropriate and up-to-date information and are of a good condition. Strangely, signs and posters often disappear on a regular basis at reception and elsewhere in the clinic. Alternatively, you may feel the need to adopt a 'mystery patient' approach. This involves arranging for someone to attend the practice and provide confidential feedback on what it was like from their perspective. If this was done by someone with a disability they could inform you not only about whether their confidentiality was maintained and whether they were treated with dignity and respect, but also about wider issues such as physical access and the provision of information. This is just one of the many approaches that you can take in investigating patient experiences.

The following scenario demonstrates how clinical audit can benefit practice.

> As senior practice nurse, nurse T had an interest in improving practice and ensuring that it was evidence based. She had instigated an audit to examine the amount of wound swabs taken and the levels of wound infection.
>
> The practice had clear 'best practice statements' that wounds should be swabbed only if signs of infection were present and also for the treatment of wounds and on the principles of cross-infection.
>
> Over the previous 12 months both the number of wound swabs taken and infection levels had dropped. These figures were collected 3 monthly. At the following reaudit it appeared that the number of swabs taken had more than doubled and infection rates had increased but not so dramatically.
>
> Nurse T realised that during this time period the only real change within the surgery was that a new practice nurse had started. Re-examining the figures in more detail showed that she was swabbing all wounds routinely and that many of the patients who had developed infections had been treated more or less exclusively by this new nurse.
>
> This identified several training needs that nurse T was able to facilitate.

Q12.9 What is meant by investigating patient experiences?

For many years patients have been seen as passive recipients of heath care, but increasingly the move is towards partnership in care, where patients have an active role and responsibility in decision-making and care management. When you are reviewing the quality of the care you provide, one of the key aspects of this is to reflect on the patient's experiences. Some information would be available from patient complaints and comments as discussed previously, but if you were looking for specific information about management of wound care you would probably have to consider taking a more positive approach to finding out what people think about the care that you are offering. The main approaches to this are postal or other surveys, face-to-face or phone semi-structured interviews or focus groups. There are various strengths and weaknesses attached to all of these, which you need to consider before deciding on the best way forward.

The first question that you need to consider before embarking on any of these techniques is Q12.10.

Q12.10 What am I going to do with the results?

You need to be clear in your own mind what questions you feel need answering and what you will do with the answers, from both technical and service delivery points of view. Undertaking a large-scale survey of everyone who lives in your clinical area would be very expensive in terms of both time and resources. Even before you had any results back, you would need to develop and pilot questionnaires, get them printed and distributed, and then you would have to think about what you would do with the results, including data input and analysis. You might think that it would be easier to hold a focus group or interview some patients, but again you need to think through all the implications such as preparing interview schedules, time to arrange and undertake the interviews, and how you are going to collate and use the results. Other issues that you need to consider are ethical ones. There is no point asking patients if they would prefer to be treated in the back room of the local pub if you know the landlord is terrified by mention of all things medical and faints at the sight of a stethoscope. More seriously you would need to consider the implications of unmet needs or desires. You may feel that getting patients to talk about wanting treatments that are not funded by your health authority raises unrealistic expectations; alternatively starting to quantify and explore such demands may help inform of such decisions. Before embarking on a patient consultation or participation exercise, you need to think through what support and resources you have to compile, disseminate and action the results of your work. This may include gaining access to computers and skills in managing information, spreadsheets and databases. You will require commitment from all the practice staff to discuss and consider any issues raised seriously and you will need to decide how feedback and changes could best be provided for the patients themselves. Your local Community Health Council (CHC), an independent organisation appointed to support patient empowerment within the NHS, may be able to advise and support you in seeking the views of your patients.

Q12.11 What sort of questions should be asked?

Before deciding on the best approach to use in finding out patient views, it is worthwhile thinking about what it is you want to know. You might want to collect statistics on the prevalence of side effects, whether specific information was provided or on what other health services were accessed by the patient. These can be established by asking what are referred to as 'closed questions', i.e. a question with yes/no or a limited number of possible responses. Examples include:

- How often is the dressing changed on your wound?
- Have you had one or more episodes of wound infection?
- Do you see a hospital consultant about your wound?

In research terms these questions provide information that is quantitative in nature; it answers the 'how' questions, looking at issues such as 'how many?', 'how often?' and 'how much?' The other sorts of information that you are likely to want to collect relate to qualitative research. Qualitative research addresses the 'why?' and 'what?' questions, the softer information that explains why people do the things that cannot be counted in figures. Examples of these sorts of questions can include:

- What do you feel has been good about the care that you have received?
- What could have been done differently to provide better standards of care?
- In what ways have you had to change your lifestyle because of your leg ulcer?

These questions can often be used to explore the statistical data in a little more depth, e.g. you might wish to explore what people feel are the advantages and disadvantages of coming to the practice for treatment rather than being seen in their own home. You will probably find that you want a variety of qualitative and quantitative information. In asking patients about their experience of wound care, you might want to know both quantitative information, about how long they have had their wound and how many days it has caused them to miss work, as well as qualitative information including how they would describe the pain they had experienced and what their experiences were of accessing care.

> Q12.12 What are the advantages and disadvantages of undertaking a patient survey?

Patient surveys are generally handed out to patients or sent to them at home with a freepost envelope for them to return their responses. They can be quite useful for finding out how many people have opinions and feelings about particular issues and are most effective when consisting of mostly yes/no and multiple choice answers. Response rates are improved if the questionnaires are relatively short (a maximum of four sides of A4 paper, preferably two sides) and are relevant to the people answering them, e.g. you are likely to get a lower response to about how people feel about the practice than you are to a more specific survey about how people feel about the management of their leg ulcer or post-surgical wound. Response rates for general surveys are notoriously low and often less than 30% are returned. It is better to avoid open-ended questions as far as possible because people do not like spending time providing lengthy written responses and the results of these are difficult to collate. Surveys like this can be most useful when you have identified a particular issue or concern, perhaps as a result of a focus group or through patient complaints or staff concerns, and you are anxious to see how widespread the feelings are among the practice population. One issue you would need to consider would be whether your target population could read and write English to a specifically high standard to be able to participate in the survey. You may need to get the questions and responses translated or adopt alternative approaches to gaining patient views.

Q12.13Have you any thoughts about interviews and focus groups?

The usefulness of interviews and focus groups principally lies in the opportunity to explore feelings about and experiences of service delivery in more depth than that allowed by a written survey. Rather than having a series of set questions with a small range of answers you would use a semi-structured questionnaire that focuses on more open-ended responses and allows participants to expand on the issues that they found of particular concern. Focus groups generally consist of four to ten people who have experienced a particular service, and through sharing their experiences they often spark ideas off each other and can help to identify particular themes. This can be particularly helpful if you are looking for suggestions about ways of improving or changing service delivery. These groups can be held either in the surgery or at a 'neutral' venue.

Interviews are generally held on a one-to-one basis, occasionally with the participant being accompanied by a friend or relative and the interviewer being accompanied by someone who takes notes on the discussion. They can be held in any venue of the interviewee's choosing and so can be particularly good for discovering the views about mobility problems or from those whose conditions are such that they do not feel like discussing them in front of a large group of people. One issue to bear in mind is that people often feel uncomfortable when talking about the care they have received with the person who actually provided that care. People do not generally like telling someone that they were not happy with what they did and may feel that their future care could be prejudiced. You may feel that it would be better to get someone who is less involved with direct patient care to undertake the interview or focus group, maybe a practice manager or someone suggested by your local clinical governance lead or a practice nurse from another practice, or community nurse manager or colleague.

There are various approaches to enlisting participants for these interviews. You may choose to put up posters in the waiting room and then wait to see who attends, although this can be a soul-destroying exercise as you may find yourself alone in the room. Alternatively, you could use the meeting of an existing user group or patient council to elicit their views. You may target a particular group of patients and write inviting them to participate, explaining what the meeting is likely to include and how long it is likely to take and providing them with a tear-off slip for them to indicate whether they wish to participate. The response may also indicate needs for interpreters or disabled access. In setting up the group, you would also need to consider issues of language needs, transportation, refreshments and childcare facilities.

The general pattern to such interviews or groups is to start by explaining the purpose of the meeting and to clarify that the participants understand and consent to this. This is often the time that permission is gained to tape-record the interview. If you decide not to record the interviews or groups, you would need to arrange for a colleague to take extensive notes on the proceedings because it is virtually impossible to facilitate the conversation and record it simultaneously. You will need to reassure the participants that, although their comments are recorded, they will be treated with confidentiality and that they will not be personally identified in any subsequent reports. The first questions generally aim to be non-controversial to allow people to get used to talking without feeling that they have to reveal too much too soon. This can include questions such as:

How long have you had your leg ulcer and where have you received care for it?

This then leads to more personal questions about what people have found helpful about their care and what could have been done differently. With a focus group the idea is to allow participants to talk among themselves, although not to the extent that they form splinter groups, and for them to share their experiences with each other as well as with you. Even if your concerns are focused on a particular issue such as waiting times, you should allow time for participants to express their views on other aspects of their care and treatment.

When closing the interview or focus group, you need to thank the members for their time and participation and explain what will happen next. You should tell people what you are going to do with their comments and the results of the project, and how you are going to let them and other patients know what you have done. This may include sending them copies of any reports and action plans, plus putting up posters in the practice and inviting them to the opening of any new services that were in part the results of their comments.

Q12.14 What else can be done to ensure that patient views are taken on board?

Staff working in primary care often have the closest links to the health needs and experiences of the local community. This was part of the driving force of the establishment of PCGs and the changes in the NHS, and puts the community nurse in a key position to help ensure that service delivery is sensitive to local needs. Patient comments and complaints can be key in assisting in this process. Although a patient complaint is often experienced as a negative experience or as a breakdown in communication, it can also offer a real opportunity to the primary care team. By reflecting on what has gone wrong in the past we can start to address policies and procedures to help ensure that similar difficulties do not arise in the future. Many complaints arise from lack of communication and may help stimulate you to think about how you can best relate to your local population, whether through conversation, demonstration of techniques, leaflets, book lists, or even cassettes and videos in a variety of languages. By starting to tap into local concerns you can start to tackle the issues that are faced at the coal front, a unique set of circumstances and conditions experienced at local level.

Rather than think about complaints as a negative thing to be avoided and diverted at all costs, you could start to think more creatively about how patients can share their experiences, comments, compliments and concerns with you and your team. One of the simplest ways of doing this is by setting up a comments box within the surgery or clinic, perhaps accompanied by a wipe board on which you could highlight issues raised and what you have done about them. You may find that the number of complaints received by the practice actually reduce as patients can share their concerns before they reach that level of severity. One of the other effects that you are likely to experience is the encouragement derived from positive comments and experiences. Many patients welcome the opportunity to say thank you and to comment on what they have found helpful, and you can further develop your strengths by reflecting on these remarks.

Q12.15 What is reflective practice and critical incident analysis?

Reflective practice and critical incident analysis are techniques that can help the individual reflect on the care received by individual patients. Critical incidence analysis often takes place within multidisciplinary groups of staff when particular patients who had exceptional outcomes, whether good or ill, are discussed. These may include unexpected deaths, avoidable amputation, violence against staff or other patients, areas where care is suspected to be less than optimum and patients with exceptionally good outcomes. All members of staff could be encouraged to identify such cases from which lessons could be learned by the team as a whole. In tracking what happened to an individual patient, you may be able to identify delays in treatment, problems with communication and possible training needs. The aim of such groups is not to be judgemental but to encourage ongoing learning in all members of the team on a permanent basis.

It is also useful to undertake reflective practice as an individual practitioner by thinking about what has happened to a particular patient. You should be able to identify what worked well and where things could be improved to help inform the future care of similar patients. Many staff keep a reflective practice diary as part of their ongoing development portfolio and use it to think through issues in relation to individual patients such as:

- What were you expecting to happen with this patient?
- What was your role in the patient's care?
- What happened that you expected to happen?
- What happened that you did not predict?
- How do you feel about what happened?
- How do you feel about your role in what happened?
- What do you think could have been done differently?
- What have you learnt from what happened?
- What might you do if a similar situation arose again?
- What are the pros and cons of different options?
- What outcomes would you look for?

Such records can help you to record your successes, personal development and learning, feelings and moods, insights and questions. They can also be as a basis for seeking feedback from colleagues about their perceptions of the same incidents and to integrate on- and off-site learning and training needs.

Q12.16 There seems to be so much to do in evaluating the care provided to the patients. Where do I start?

Don't feel that you have to do everything all of the time. It is probably a good idea to focus on a particular area of care such as the management of leg ulcers. Then get hold of the *Effective Health Care Bulletin* and any other evidence you can find and audit a few sets of case notes to see how you are doing. Decide on how you are going to approach a few patients to see how they feel about the care you provide. Just as you reflect on the care you have provided to individual patients, reflect on what works and what doesn't in evaluating care. You may find that no one responds to a comments box or that people don't like coming out at night to attend a focus group. In that case you may need to try alternative approaches, such as interviews at home or securing a tape-recorder in the waiting room so that people can leave their views as sound bites. Remember this process is not meant to be threatening; don't just focus on the negative. Take time to enjoy and reflect on the positive comments and compliments that you have received. These tools can help you to do an even better job and to give you the satisfaction of ongoing development and refinement of your own skills and ability.

Summary

By developing your skills in evidence-based health care you can help to ensure that you are providing up-to-date and effective care for your patients. Clinical audit is a tool to help you review care systematically and ensure that you have implemented standards for best practice. Patients are key informants and participants in care and there are a variety of approaches that can be used to reflect on their opinions on the care that they have received. Complaints should be viewed as valuable opportunities to learn from patient experiences and improve the care provided by the practice. By reflecting on individual patient cases, you can identify areas of good practice, training and learning needs, and make changes to practice processes that can affect the care of the whole practice population.

Glossary

Abscess: a localised collection of necrotic tissue, bacteria and white cells, known as pus contained in a capsule, the wall of which is formed from phagocytes and strands of fibrin (see Q6.5).

Albumin: a soluble protein which is a major component of serum proteins (see Q3.4).

Anaerobe: bacteria that do not tolerate free oxygen from the air, and grow where there is either no air or there are low levels of oxygen (see Q2.7).

Anaerobic: conditions with a lack of oxygen (see Q 5.6).

Angiogenesis: the formation of new blood vessels at the base of a wound; this occurs during the proliferative phase of healing (see Q1.8).

Ankle brachial pressure index (ABPI): the result of a Doppler ultra-sonography test used to determine the presence and level of arterial disease in patients with leg ulcers (see Q8.12).

Ankle flare: associated with venous disease of the leg. Small vessels distend and appear around the ankle and heel (see Q8.4).

Atherosclerosis: a disease of the arterial wall in which the inner layer thickens causing a narrowing and hardening of the vessels (see Q8.15).

Autolysis: the breakdown of devitalised tissue by leukocytes (see Q1.8).

Cellulitis: a spreading infection of the soft tissue, which is characterised by redness, heat, oedema and pain (see Q10.5).

Collagen: a protein substance, which provides fibres that make up the supportive network of connective tissue. Produced during the proliferative stage of wound healing and remodelled during the maturation phase (see Q1.8).

Colonisation: multiplication of micro-organisms without provoking a corresponding host reaction (see Q10.1).

Commensals: non-pathogenic micro-organisms that do not react with their host and become part of the normal body flora (see Q10.1).

Contamination: presence of micro-organisms (such as commensals) without multiplication (see Q10.1).

Contraction: wounds that have granulated start to contract, drawing the edges towards each other and reducing the surface of the raw area (see Q1.8).

Débridement: the removal of foreign material and devitalised tissue from a wound until surrounding healthy tissue is exposed (see Q2.10).

Dehiscence: the breakdown of a closed wound resulting in an open wound.

Devitalise: to deprive of vitality or life.

Doppler ultrasonography: used to record the ankle brachial pressure index by detecting the blood flow in the peripheral arteries (see Q8.12).

Epithelialisation: the final stage of the proliferative stage of healing when the wound surface becomes covered with epithelium (see Q1.8).

Epithelium/epithelial tissue: the tissue covering the surface of the body, lining body cavities and forming glands (see Q1.8).

Erythema: redness of the skin produced by congestion of the capillaries (see Q1.8).

Eschar: a scab consisting of dried serum and devitalised dermal cells, which covers damage caused by a burn, abrasion, ulcers or other skin disease, defect or infection (see Q2.10).

Excoriation: damage to the surface of the skin caused by physical abrasion such as scratching or dragging the patients over sheets (see Q9.5).

Extrinsic: operating from the outside, not originating in the body part in question (see Q9.3).

Exudate: the fluid formed at the surface of a wound as a result of small vessels leaking into the wound. Contains protein and cells (see Q1.8 and Q11.5).

Fibrin: an insoluble elastic protein derived from fibrinogen. Involved in the clotting mechanism (see Q1.8).

Granulation: the formation of new tissue which fills the wound during the proliferative stage of healing (see Q1.8 and Q2.12).

Haematoma: a collection of blood in the tissues.

Haemostasis: process leading to the reduction of blood loss from the body (see Q1.8).

Healing by primary (first) intention: closed wounds with a minor defect (see Q1.7).

Healing by secondary intention: open wounds allowed to heal by granulation (see Q1.7).

Healing by tertiary intention: wound initially left open to drain and surgically closed at a later date (see Q1.7).

Infection: multiplication of micro-organisms producing a host reaction (see Chapter 10).

Inflammation: initial response of the body after injury (see Q1.8).

Ischaemia: localised deficiency of blood and therefore oxygen, caused by obstruction of the blood vessels (see Q2.10 and Q8.15).

Keloid: a protuberance of progressively enlarging scar tissue, caused by excessive collagen, which may extend into normal tissue (see Q7.7).

Lipodermatosclerosis: brown staining of the lower leg occurring as a result of haemoglobin breakdown, closely associated with venous hypertension and ulceration (see Q8.4).

Maceration: softening or sogginess of the tissues resulting from the retention of excessive moisture (see Q11.5).

Macrophage: phagocytic cell which plays a vital role in inflammation and initiates angiogenesis (see Q1.8).

Maturation stage: the final stage of wound healing (see Q1.8).

Necrosis: localised tissue death. Usually black or brown in colour (see Q2.10. and Q8.15).

Neutrophil: a white blood cell which ingests bacteria (see Q1.8).

Occlusive dressing: a dressing that totally covers a wound, sealing it off from the environment (see Q5.6).

Oedema: excess tissue fluid (see Q1.8. and Q8.6).

Osteomyelitis: infection of bone.

Overgranulation (hypergranulation): granulation tissue which is raised above the level of the wound (see Q11.6).

Phagocytosis: the process of engulfing micro-organisms, foreign cells and debris by macrophages or neutrophils (see Q1.8).

Platelet: component of blood. Involved in the inflammatory stage of healing (see Q1.8).

Pus: fluid consisting of exudate, dead and exhausted macrophages and bacteria (see Q6.5).

Scab: see Eschar.

Septicaemia: systemic disease. Pathogenic micro-organisms or other toxins are present and persist in the bloodstream (see Q10.4).

Skin graft: skin is removed from its normal location and used to cover another open area (see Q7.6).

Slough: devitalised tissue which is yellow, cream or grey in colour (see Q2.11).

Toxin: substance having a detrimental (toxic) effect on living cells.

Ulcer: a persistent area of discontinuity of the epidermis and dermis (see Q8.1).

Vasculitis: inflammation of small arteries or veins with resulting fibrosis and thrombus formation. Often associated with rheumatoid disease (see Q8.16).

Venous hypertension: abnormally high pressure in the venous system (see Q8.4).

Resources

Convatec (wound care helpline)
Tel: 0800 289738

Credenhill Limited
10 Cossall Industrial Estate
Ilkeston
Derbyshire DE7 5UG
Tel: 0115 932 0144
Fax: 0115 944 0437
Email: sales@credenhill.co.uk
Made-to-measure compression hosiery on NHS prescription.

European Pressure Ulcer Advisory Panel
EPUAP Business Office
Wound healing unit
Department of Dermatology
Churchill Hospital
Old Road
Headington, Oxford OX3 7LJ
Tel: 01865 228269
Fax: 01865 228233
Email: EuropeanPressureUlcerAdvisPanel@compuserve.com

SCAR information service
PO Box 2003
Hull HU3 4DJ
Tel: 0845 120 00 22
Website: www.carinfo.org
Information on scarring treatments and support organisations.

Smith & Nephew (wound care helpline)
Tel: 0800 590173

Tissue Viability Society
Glanville Centre
Salisbury
Wiltshire SP2 8BJ
Tel: 01722 429057
Fax: 01722 425263
Email: tvs@dial,pipex.com
Website: www.tvs.org.uk

The Waterlow Pressure Sore Prevention/Treatment Policy

Judy Waterlow
Newtons
Curland
Taunton TA3 5SG
Information on the use of Waterlow and other pressure sore prevention techniques.

The Wound Care Society
Mrs Hazel Morley
PO Box 170
Huntingdon PE18 7PL
Tel: 01480 434401
Email: wound.care.society@talk21.com
Website: www.woundcaresociety.org
Information about all aspects of wound management.

Websites

Dermatological issues

www.skinsite.com

Wound care with educational basis

www.medicaledu.com

Abstracts, articles, product links and industry news

www.woundcarenet.com

Free registration – includes microbiology, case studies, trials and larval therapy

www.medscape.com

Wound care using aromatherapy

www.alternativemedicine.com

General wound care forum

www.wound.net

Connection to all of these sites can be made at:

www.masltd.co.uk

References

Ackroyd JS, Young AE (1983) Leg ulcers that do not heal. *British Medical Journal* **286**: 207–208.

Angeras MH, Brandenberg A, Falk A, Seeman T (1991) Comparison between sterile saline and tap water for the cleansing of acute traumatic soft tissue wounds. *European Journal of Surgery* **158**(33): 347–350.

Armstrong M (1998) Obesity as an intrinsic factor affecting wound healing. *Journal of Wound Care* **7**(5): 220–221.

Ashford RF, Plant GT, Maher J (1984) Double blind trial of metronidazole in malodorous ulcerating tumours. Lancet **i**: 1232–1233.

Asquith S (1999) The use of aromatherapy in wound care. *Journal of Wound Care* **8**(6): 318–320.

Banks V (1997) Pressure sore education. *Journal of Wound Care* **6**(10): 506–507.

Barnhorst DA, Barner HB (1968) Prevalence of congenitally absent foot pulses. *New England Journal of Medicine* **278**: 264–265.

Barrett E (1987) Putting risk calculators in their place. *Nursing Times* **83**(7): 65–70.

Bellamy K (1995) Photography in wound assessment. *Journal of Wound Care* **4**(7): 313–316.

Bennett L, Lee BY (1986) Pressure versus shear in pressure sore formation. In: Lee BY, ed. *Chronic Ulcers of the Skin*. New York: McGraw-Hill, pp. 39–55.

Birchall L (1993) Making sense of pressure sore prediction calculators. *Nursing Times* **89**(18): 34–37.

Black D (1982) *Inequalities in Health (Black Report)*. Harmondsworth: Penguin.

Bland KI, Plain WE, von Fraunhofer JA (1984) Experimental and clinical observations of the effects of cytotoxic chemotherapeutic drugs on wound healing. *Annals of Surgery* **199**: 782–790.

Bond MR (1984) *Pain: Its nature, analysis and treatment*. Edinburgh: Churchill Livingstone.

Bux M, Baig MK, Rodrigues E, Armstrong D, Brown A (1997) Antibody response to topical streptokinase. *Journal of Wound Care* **6**(2): 70–73.

Cameron J (1998) Skin care for patients with chronic leg ulcers. *Journal of Wound Care* **7**(9): 459–462.

Charles H (1999) Short stretch bandages in the treatment of venous leg ulcers. *Journal of Wound Care* **8**(6): 303–304.

Cherry GW, Ryan TJ (1985) Enhanced wound angiogenesis with a new hydrocolloid dressing. In: Ryan TJ, ed. *An Environment for Healing. The role of occlusion*. International Congress and Symposium. Series no. 88. London: Royal Society of Medicine.

Choiniere M, Melzack R, Girand N (1990) Comparisons between patient and nurses assessment of pain and medication efficacy in severe burn injuries. *Pain* **40**: 143–152.

Chrintz H (1989) Need for surgical wound dressings. *British Journal of Surgery* **76**: 204–205.

Clark M, Fletcher J (1999) Product selection. Resource file. Mattresses and beds. *Journal of Wound Care* (suppl 4): 1–8.

Closs JS (1993) Malnutrition. The key to pressure sores? *Nursing Standard* **8**(4): 32–36.

Collier M (1999a) Mattresses and beds. Part 1. *Journal of Wound Care* (suppl 8): 7.

Collier M (1999b) Pressure ulcer development and principles for prevention. In: Miller M, Glover D, eds. *Wound Management Theory and Practice*. London: Nursing Times Books.

Cooper DM (1990) Optimising wound healing. *Nursing Clinics of North America* **25**(1): 165.

Cooper R, Lawrence JC (1996) The isolation and identification of bacteria from wounds. *Journal of Wound Care* **5**(7): 335–340.

Cutting KF (1999) Factors influencing wound healing. *Nursing Standard* **8**(50): 33–36.

Cutting KF, Harding KG (1994) Criteria for identifying wound infection. *Journal of Wound Care* **3**(4): 198–201.

David J (1986) *Wound Management. A comprehensive guide to dressing and healing*. London: Martin Dunitz.

Davies K (1994) Pressure sores: aetiology, risk factors and assessment scales. *British Journal of Nursing* **3**(6): 256–260.

Dealey C (1993) Measuring the prevalence and incidence of pressure sores. *British Journal of Nursing* **2**(20): 998–1006.

Dealey C (1994) *The Care of Wounds: A guide for nurses*. Oxford: Blackwell Scientific Publications.

Dealey C (1995) Pressure sores and incontinence: a study evaluating the use of topical agents in skin care. *Journal of Wound Management* **4**(3): 103–105.

Department of Health (1991) *Dietary Reference Values for Food, Energy and Nutrients for the UK*. (Report on Health and Social Subjects no. 41) London: HMSO.

Dickerson JWT (1993) Ascorbic acid, zinc and wound healing. *Journal of Wound Care* **2**(6): 350–353.

Draper J (1985) Making the dressing fit the wound. *Nursing Times* **81**(4): 32–35.

Duckworth GJ (1990) Revised guidelines for the control of epidemic methicillin resistant *Staphylococcus aureus*. *Journal of Hospital Infection* **16**: 351–377.

Dyson M, Young S, Pendle C (1988) Comparison of the effects of moist and dry conditions on dermal repair. *Journal of Investigative Dermatology* **91**(5): 435–449.

Effective Health Care Bulletin (1995) Nuffield Institute for Health. University of Leeds. NHS Centre for Reviews and Dissemination. University of York.

Ek AC, Boman G (1982) A descriptive study of pressure sores: the prevalence of pressure sores and characteristics of patients. *Journal of Advanced Nursing* **7**: 51–57.

Emflorgo CA (1998) Letters. *Journal of Wound Care* **7**(5): 235.

Emflorgo CA (1999) The assessment of wound pain. *Journal of Wound Care* **8**(8): 384–385.

European Pressure Ulcer Advisory Panel (EPUAP) (1997) *Pressure Ulcer Treatment Guidelines*. Oxford: EPUAP.

Flanagan M (1993) Predicting pressure sore risk. *Journal of Wound Care* **2**(4): 215–218.

Fletcher A (1992) The epidemiology of two common age related wounds. *Journal of Wound Care* **1**(4): 39–43.

Fletcher J (1999) A practical approach to dressing wounds in difficult positions. *British Journal of Nursing* **8**(12): 779–786.

Fowler A, Dempsey A (1998) Split thickness skin donor sites. *Journal of Wound Care* **7**(8): 399–402.

Gardner AMN, Fox RH (1986) The return of blood to the heart against the force of gravity. In: Negus D, Jantet G, eds. *Phlebology*. London: Libby, pp. 65–67.

Gould D (1997) Pilonidal sinus. *Nursing Times* **93**(suppl): 32.

Gower JP, Lawrence JC (1995) The incidence, causes and treatment of minor burns. *Journal of Wound Care* **4**(2): 71–74.

Green C (1993) Antistreptokinase titres after topical streptokinase. *Lancet* **341**: 1602–1603.

Grey JE (1998) Cellulitis associated with wounds. *Journal of Wound Care* **7**(7): 338–340.

Groscott P (1995) The palliative management of fungating malignant wounds. *Journal of Wound Care* **4**(5): 240–242.

Guest G, Pearson S (1997) Recovery on a plate. *Nursing Times* **93**(46): 84–86.

Hodgkin W (1998) Pilonidal sinus disease. *Journal of Wound Care* **7**(9): 481–483.

Hofman D, Ryan T, Arnold F (1997) Pain in venous leg ulcers. *Journal of Wound Care* **6**(5): 222–224.

Hoskins J, Welchew M (1985) *Post-operative Pain. Understanding its nature and how to treat it.* London: Faber & Faber.

Hutchinson JJ, Lawrence JC (1991) Wound infection under occlusive dressings. *Journal of Hospital Infection* **17**: 83–84.

Johnson A (1988) Wound management. Are you getting it right? *Professional Nurse* **3**(8): 306–309.

Joseph WS, Axler DA (1990) Microbiology and antimicrobial therapy of diabetic foot infections. *Clinics in Podiatric Medicine and Surgery* **7**(3): 467–481.

Kendrick M, Lucker K, Cullun N, Roe B (1994) *Clinical Information Pack*. Number 1. *The management of leg ulcers in the community*. University of Liverpool.

Kenney L, Rithalia S (1999) Technical aspects of support surfaces. Mattresses and beds. Resource file. *Journal of Wound Care* (suppl part 3): 1–8.

Land L (1994) *A Review of Pressure Damage Prevention Strategies*. A report initiated by West Midlands Regional Health Authority.

Lawrence JC (1996) First aid measures for the treatment of burns and scalds. *Journal of Wound Care* **5**(7): 319–322.

Lawrence JC (1997) Wound irrigation. *Journal of Wound Care* **6**(1): 23–26.

Levin ME (1988) The diabetic foot: pathophysiology, evaluation and treatment. In Levin ME, O'Neal LW, eds. *The Diabetic Foot*, 4th edn. St Louis: CV Mosby, pp. 1–15.

Lewis BK (1998) Nutritional intake and the risk of pressure sore development in the older patient. *Journal of Wound Care* **7**(1): 31–35.

Loader S, Delue M, Hoffman D (1994) A constancy service that pays dividends, setting up a pressure service relief group. *Professional Nurse* **10**: 259–266.

Lock PM (1980) The effect of temperature on mitotic activity at the edge of experimental wounds. In: Lundgren A, Soner AB, eds. *Symposia on Wound Healing: Plastic, surgical and dermatological aspects*. Sweden: Molndal.

Lothian P, Barbenal J, eds (1983) *Nursing Aspects of Pressure Sore Development in Pressure Sores*. London: Macmillan.

McCaffery M (1983) *Nursing the Patient in Pain*. London: Harper & Row.

McLaren SMG (1992) Nutrition and wound healing. *Journal of Wound Care* **1**(3): 45–55.

McLeod A (1997) Principles of alternating pressure surfaces. *Advances in Wound Care* **10**: 30–36.

Makleburst J, Siegreen M (1996) *Pressure Ulcers. Guidelines for prevention and nursing management*, 2nd edn. Springhouse, PA: Springhouse Corporation.

Miller M (1995) Wound care for minor injuries. *Primary Health Care* **5**(10): 23–26.

Miller M (1999) Wound assessment. In: Miller M, Glover D, eds. *Wound Management, Theory and Practice*. London: Nursing Times Books.

Miller M, Dyson M (1996) *The Principles of Wound Care*. London: Macmillan Magazines Ltd.

Moffatt C (1998) Issues in the assessment of leg ulceration. *Journal of Wound Care* **7**(9): 469–473.

Moffatt C, O'Hare L (1995) Graduated compression hosiery for venous ulceration. *Journal of Wound Care* **4**(10): 459–462.

Moody M (1993) Accountability in wound care: a practical approach. *Wound Management* **3**(1): 6–7.

Morgan D (1987) *Formulary of Wound Management Products*. Cardiff: Whitchurch Hospital.

Morgan D (1994) *Formulary of Wound Management Products*, 6th edn. Haselmere: Euromed Communications.

Morgan D (1997) *Formulary of Wound Management Products*, 7th edn. Haselmere: Euromed Communications.

Morison M (1989) Pressure sores: removing the cause of the wound. *Professional Nurse* **5**: 97–104.

Morison M (1991) *A Colour Guide to the Assessment and Management of Leg Ulcers*. London: Wolfe Publishing Ltd.

Morison M, Moffatt C (1994) *A Colour Guide to the Assessment and Management of Leg Ulcers*, 2nd edn. London: Mosby, Times Mirror International Publishers Ltd.

Mortimer P (1993) Skin problems in palliative care: medical aspects. In: Doyle D, Hanks G, Macdonald N, eds. *Oxford Textbook of Palliative Medicine*. Oxford: Oxford Medical Publications.

Mosely JG (1988) *Palliation in Malignant Disease*. Edinburgh: Churchill Livingstone.

Myers JA (1982) Wound healing and the use of a modern surgical dressing. *The Pharmaceutical Journal* **229**(6186): 103–104.

Newman V, Allwood M, Oakes R (1989) The use of metronidazole gel to control the smell of malodorous lesions. *Palliative Medicine* **3**(4): 303–305.

NHS Executive (1995) *Consensus Strategy For Management of Leg Ulcers*. Leeds: NHS Executive.

North Thames Research Appraisal Group (1998) *The Clinical Effectiveness Process*. London: NTRAG.

Norton D, McLaren R, Exton Smith AN (1962) *Investigations of Geriatric Nursing Problems in Hospital*. Edinburgh: Churchill Livingstone.

Nyquist R, Hawthorne PJ (1987) The prevalence of pressure sores in a Health Authority. *Journal of Advanced Nursing* **12**: 183–187.

Parker LJ (1999) Importance of hand washing in reducing cross infection. *British Journal of Nursing* **8**: 716–720.

Partridge C (1998) Influential factors in surgical wound healing. *Journal of Wound Care* **7**(7): 350–353.

Pitcher M (1998) Internet sources on leg ulcer management. *Journal of Wound Care* **7**(6): 313–316.

Plewa M (1990) Altered host response and special infections in the elderly. *Emergency Medicine Clinics in North America* **8**(2): 93–206.

Priest C, Clarke M (1993) Update: pressure sore risk factors. *Journal of Wound Care* **2**(4): 216–217.

Professional Development (1994) Wound care. Knowledge for practice. *Nursing Times* **90**: 49.

Pun YLW, Barraclough DRE, Muirden KD (1990) Leg ulcers in rheumatoid arthritis. *Medical Journal of Australia* **153**(10): 585–587.

Reid J, Morison M (1994) Towards a consensus classification of pressure sores. *Journal of Wound Care* **3**(3): 293–294.

Saxey S (1986) The nurses response to postoperative pain. *Nursing* **3**(10): 377–381.

Seers K (1987) Perceptions of pain. *Nursing Times* **83**(48): 37–38.

Silver IA (1985) Oxygen and tissue repair In: Ryan TJ, ed. *An Environment for Healing. The role of occlusion*. International Congress and Symposium. Series no. 88. London: Royal Society of Medicine.

Silver J (1987) Letter. *Care Science and Practice* **5**: 30.

Staas WE, Cioschi HM (1991) Pressure sores – a multifaceted approach to prevention and treatment. Rehabilitation medicine. *Western Journal of Medicine* **154**: 539–544.

Stevens J (1998) Letters. *Journal of Wound Care* **7**(5): 235.

Thomas S (1990) *Wound Management and Dressings*. London: The Pharmaceutical Press.

Thomas S (1998) The importance of secondary dressings in wound care. *Journal of Wound Care* **7**(4): 189–192.

Thomas S, Jones M, Shutter S, Andrews A (1996) Reader questions. *Journal of Wound Care Nursing* **92**: 46.

Thomas S, Vowden K (1998) Readers' questions. *Journal of Wound Care* **7**(3): 154.

Thompson PD, Smith DJ (1994) What is infection? *American Journal of Surgery* **67a**(suppl): 75–115.

Torrance C (1983) *Pressure Sores: Aetiology, treatment and prevention*. London: Croom Helm.

Turner TD (1985) Which dressing and why? In: Wesby S, ed. *Wound Care*. London: William Heinemann Medical Books.

United Kingdom Central Council (1992) *Code of Professional Conduct*. London: UKCC.

Value for Money Unit (1997) *A Prescribers' Guide to Dressings and Wound Management Materials*. Report produced with *Journal of Wound Care*.

Vowden KR, Goulding V, Vowden P (1996) Hand held Doppler assessment for peripheral arterial disease. *Journal of Wound Care* **5**(3): 125–128.

Warfield CA (1997) *Expert Pain Management*. Springhouse, PA: Springhouse Corporation.

Waterlow J (1985) A risk assessment card. *Nursing Times* **81**(48): 49–55.

Weaver A (1996) MRSA and its management in the community. *Community Nurse* **2**(9): 36–38.

West P, Priestley J (1994) Money under the mattress. *Health Service Journal* **14**: 20–22.

Williams C (1999) An investigation into the benefits of Aquacel Hydrofibre wound dressing. *British Journal of Nursing* **8**(10): 676–680.

Williams E (1997) Assessing the future. *Nursing Times* **93**(suppl): 23.

Winter G (1962) Formation of the scab and the rate of epithelialization of superficial wounds in the skin of the young domestic pig. *Nature* **193**: 293–294.

Wolverhampton Health Care Control of Infection Committee (WHC CIC) (1995) *Methicillin Resistant* Staphylococcus aureus *Policy*. Wolverhampton: WHC CIC.

The Wound Programme (1992) Centre for Medical Education, University of Dundee, Scotland.

Index

Page references in **bold type** refer to
definitions of terms in the Glossary